I Need an
Operation...
Now What?

A Pat͗   Guide to a Safe
ar ͗   ͗ssful Outcome

Thomas R. Russell, MD, FACS
Executive Director, American College of Surgeons

Thomson Healthcare

THOMSON

The information and advice in this book are based on the training, personal experiences, and research of the author. Its contents are obtained from sources the author believes to be reliable; however, the information presented is not intended to substitute for professional medical advice. The author and the publisher urge you to consult with your physician or other qualified health care provider prior to starting any treatment or undergoing any surgical procedure. Because there is always some risk involved, the author and publisher cannot be responsible for any adverse effects or consequences resulting from the use of any of the suggestions, preparations, or procedures described in this book.

ISBN 13: 978-1-56363-700-1
ISBN 10: 1-56356-700-6   MAR   2008

Printed in the United States of America

Contents

Acknowledgments, vii

Introduction, 1

1. It's All About You, 5

2. Choosing the Surgeon Who Is Best for You, 11

3. What to Ask the Surgeon at the First Meeting, 23

4. Preparing for the Operation, 35

5. Having the Operation, 49

6. After the Operation, 63

7. After You Go Home, 81

Glossary, 93

Appendix A: About the American College of Surgeons, 107

Appendix B: Surgical Specialties, 111

Appendix C: Surgical Specialty Organizations, 113

Index, 115

*Dedicated to surgical patients
and the surgeons who take care of them.*

Acknowledgments

I would like to express my sincere appreciation to all of the individuals whose efforts have made this book possible:

—To my patients, who allowed me to take care of them. It was a wonderful privilege and inspiration to have had their trust as we worked together to deal with the health issues confronting them.

—To all of my fellow surgeons, whose passionate dedication to their patients provides the impetus for continuing efforts to improve patient care.

—To all the allied health professionals who make the surgical experience a positive reality on a daily basis.

—To my surgical colleagues who took the time to review this manuscript and provide me with their invaluable insight and advice.

—To Kathleen Louden, who made the process of developing this book a far easier task than I had anticipated.

—To Linn Meyer, ACS Director of Communications, for her belief in this project and her guidance in bringing it to fruition.

And, finally, I would like to express my appreciation to the American College of Surgeons, its principles of professionalism, and its dedication to patient safety as the cornerstone of its ongoing efforts to improve surgical patient care.

Introduction

I was a practicing general surgeon for 35 years before becoming the executive director of the largest international organization of surgeons, the American College of Surgeons. In my surgical practice, I explained the process of having an operation to thousands of patients.

As an insider in the profession of surgery, I know what surgeons do, and how and why operations are performed. I decided to share my knowledge and experience through this book, which will take you behind the closed doors of the surgical process. It will give you an insider's point of view of what it's like to have an operation.

Like you, I know what it's like to be the patient. About 20 years ago, I had back pain so severe that I thought I was finished as a surgeon. It became obvious that I needed a back operation. Going into the operation, I knew that no matter how good the spine surgeon was, I had to do my part, too. I would have to work hard after the operation at exercising regularly and controlling my weight if I wanted the surgical results to last. I became an active participant in the surgical process and have had an excellent result. I also recently had a gallbladder operation and have benefited greatly from that operation.

You, too, must become an active participant in your operation. Part of the teamwork you need to have with your surgeon is to become informed about the operation you will have. Research shows that patients who are well informed about their treatment have better surgical outcomes and are more satisfied with their results.

I know what patients should ask their surgeons but often don't—because they're too afraid to ask or they don't know what to ask. In this book, I will tell you what you should ask your surgeon in order to become well informed. I'll share my experience both as a surgeon and as a patient who has had two successful operations.

NOT AN UNCOMMON LIFE EVENT

I am not alone in having been a surgical patient. Every year, between 15 and 25 million Americans undergo a surgical procedure. The chance of needing an operation at some time in your life increases after age 50. So it's likely that you or a loved one will need an operation at some point.

Having an operation is a major life event. First, the whole idea can be frightening. You face an unknown experience, in which your body is invaded and you are in a vulnerable situation. And, as your surgeon will inform you, there are risks with any surgical procedure, whether it is considered to be a major or minor procedure. Actually, there's an old saying and that is, a minor operation is one that is performed on someone else!

Even though I'm a surgical "insider," I had apprehensions before I had each of my two operations. It's okay, and even natural, to be worried or afraid about this experience, even if you are a surgeon or another health care professional.

Then, too, there is a mystique about surgery. Surgeons are shown in photos and on TV wearing masks. An operation takes place behind closed doors. No one besides the surgical team is allowed inside the operating room except the patient, who is asleep or sedated.

But having a surgical procedure can be a life-changing experience in a positive way. It can improve your health. Sometimes it even spurs you to make your lifestyle healthier. In this sense, an operation can be one of the most important events in your life.

Thus, you need to know and fully understand what it will entail and what you can expect.

WHAT'S INSIDE THIS BOOK

The goal of this book is to demystify the experience of having an operation, to make it less scary and as positive as possible. I wrote this book for you—the patient—and your family, to help you understand each step in the process of having an operation.

No matter what type of operation you are having, there are certain things that every adult patient can, and should, do before and after a surgical procedure to obtain the best chance of success. In this book, I will share with you what they are.

From time to time, you also will find my special "insider's" tip. This is helpful advice that you likely won't find in every book about having an operation.

You'll also hear from actual patients. They share how they found a surgeon, how they prepared for their operation, and what they think contributed to the success of their procedure.

And because good communication with your surgeon and the surgical team is vitally important, the end of each chapter contains a handy list of questions for your doctor. You can bring the list along to your appointment with your surgeon, so you won't forget to ask something important to you.

I Need an Operation...Now What? cannot substitute for your own research into your specific health problem and its treatment. Each surgical procedure is unique, so I cannot give you specific details about your procedure. Your surgeon can do that. Likewise, the information published in this book is not intended to take the place of a discussion with a qualified surgeon who is familiar with your situation. It is important to remember that each individual is different. The reasons for and outcomes of any operation depend on the patient's specific diagnosis, disease, or other medical condition.

What the information in this book can do is make clear the general process of having an operation. It will help you know what to expect and what to look for in a surgeon.

Even if you have had an operation in the past, you will benefit from reading this book, because surgery has changed a great deal in recent years. Thanks to minimally invasive surgical procedures, many operations that once required long hospital stays now are performed on an outpatient basis. Surgical and anesthetic techniques have advanced, and surgeons' skills are now more specialized, making operations safer and more tolerable, with a quicker recovery. Finally, surgeons no longer simply treat illness and injury. They help patients stay well and improve their quality of life.

It is my hope, and that of the American College of Surgeons, that you will use this book to deal with having an operation in an informed and confident way. The College has a long history of dedication to patient safety and providing information about surgery. With this book, we hope to make having an operation an easier experience for you. May you enjoy long-term good health.

ONE

It's All About You

- The most important things you can do to become an informed patient
- Your rights as a patient
- To operate or not to operate

Your doctor just told you that you may need a surgical procedure. You're in shock. Now what?

My advice is to take control. Become fully informed about your options. And that means asking questions.

Thirty years ago you probably would have agreed to have an operation with few questions asked. Back then most patients did not feel comfortable questioning their doctors. They often were in awe of the health care system and the surgeon. Patients relied on their physicians to make medical decisions for them and then did what the doctor told them to do. It was all about the physician and the trust the patient had in his or her doctor.

Those days are gone. Today health care is all about *you*. The patient is now an active member of the surgical team.

YOU HAVE THE RIGHT TO NOT REMAIN SILENT!

As a patient, you have rights. Under a national patients' bill of rights created in 1998 (see pages 9–10), you have the right to know all of your treatment options and to participate in decisions about your care. You also have a right to receive accurate and easily understandable information about your surgeon and other health care professionals who will be involved in your care, your health plan, and health care facilities.

Along with those and other rights, patients have responsibilities. I believe that we need to take charge of our own health. We all must be informed health care consumers as well as patients. After all, we are being asked to spend more and more of our own dollars on our health care.

You wouldn't buy a new car without first becoming an informed consumer—by finding out if it has the features you want and if the price is the best you can get. Needless to say, your body and your health are more important than what you drive. So, you need to become informed about something that affects your body and your health as much as an operation does.

Educate yourself about your medical problem and the proposed surgical procedure by researching and reading about them. There is a great deal of helpful medical information out there. Many books on health care topics are aimed at consumers. Also, many medical associations, including the American College of Surgeons, produce patient education materials and have Web sites with information about health topics. (See Appendix C on pages 113 and 114 for information on the College's Web site and for a list of surgical specialty organizations and their Web sites.) If you are unsure about the quality of information you obtain, such as from an Internet source, ask your surgeon whether the information is accurate and up-to-date.

Besides reading, talk to people you know who have had a similar operation, so you can learn what to expect.

Of course, if you need an emergency surgical procedure, you won't have time to do research. However, if your operation is planned ("elective")—and most surgical procedures are—you probably will have time to get informed. Reading this book is a great first step!

WHY DOES YOUR DOCTOR WANT YOU TO SEE A SURGEON?

Don't be afraid to ask questions of the health care provider who thinks you should see a surgeon. For starters, make sure you understand why your doctor (or physician's assistant or nurse practitioner) recommends that you see a surgeon. Ask why your condition needs a specialist's care.

If you don't understand exactly what your medical problem is, ask your doctor to explain it to you. Ask if your doctor knows the name of the operation you might need. That way you can research it before you meet with a surgeon.

DON'T BE INTIMIDATED

I encourage you to not feel intimidated when you meet with a surgeon. Part of the job of your surgeon and surgeon's staff is to inform you about your operation. Naturally, you'll have questions, even after your surgeon explains the operation. I strongly believe that patients should feel free to ask their surgeon anything they want answered about the operation or the surgeon's competency to perform it. Respectfully ask anything you want to know that will put you at ease about having a surgical procedure.

A PATIENT'S PERSPECTIVE

Amy Wells, 33-year-old who has had multiple gastrointestinal operations

"It's really easy to be intimidated by the whole surgical process. You're totally out of your element. Major surgery is scary, no matter how many times you go through it. So it's important to control what you can, by picking your surgeon and your hospital and making sure you have all the information you need to make good decisions . . . . Communication with your surgeon is so important. My surgeon asked me questions, listened to my preferences, and let me know if he could accommodate my requests."

Also, you should feel free to have a family member or friend accompany you when you meet with the surgeon. They may have questions you may not think of, and they also can ask for more information or an explanation of anything that is not clear.

Throughout this book, I emphasize the need to become informed and ask questions. However, it is possible to ask too many questions and do too much research about your operation. I had some patients who were basically drowning in information. As a result, they were often overwhelmed and unable to make a decision.

As you prepare for your operation, realize that there must be a balance between being informed and being overloaded with information.

INSIDER'S TIP

I have had patients ask me if I drank alcohol, used drugs, or was physically fit. I never was intimidated by any question. I felt that my patients had a right to know whether I was competent. As long as you ask the surgeon questions in a nonconfrontational and nonoffensive manner, you should expect an honest answer. If a surgeon is defensive about answering your questions, does not seem forthright, or is unwilling to take the time to answer your questions, you may need to look for another surgeon!

ARE THERE ALTERNATIVES TO AN OPERATION?

Ask the health care provider who is referring you to a surgeon if there are other treatment options besides an operation. These options may include nonsurgical treatments, such as medication, or a less invasive procedure.

No one really wants to have a surgical procedure. However, sometimes an operation is the best or only option for your condition, or you may need it in addition to medical treatment.

Talking to a surgeon does not necessarily mean that having a surgical procedure is inevitable. It is not uncommon for a surgeon to recommend a nonsurgical approach for your problem. A visit to a surgeon can help you decide if an operation is the right choice for you now, later, or not at all.

Remember, it's all about you.

Patients' Bill of Rights*

I. Information Disclosure

You have the right to receive accurate and easily understood information about your health plan, health care professionals, and health care facilities. If you speak another language, have a physical or mental disability, or just don't understand something, assistance will be provided so you can make informed health care decisions.

II. Choice of Providers and Plans

You have the right to a choice of health care providers that is sufficient to provide you with access to appropriate high-quality health care.

III. Access to Emergency Services

If you have severe pain, an injury, or sudden illness that convinces you that your health is in serious jeopardy, you have the right to receive screening and stabilization emergency services whenever and wherever needed, without prior authorization or financial penalty.

IV. Participation in Treatment Decisions

You have the right to know all your treatment options and to participate in decisions about your care. Parents, guardians, family members, or other individuals that you designate can represent you if you cannot make your own decisions.

---

*Adopted by the U.S. Advisory Commission on Consumer Protection and Quality in the Health Care Industry in 1998. Many health plans have adopted these principles. Source: *www.consumer.gov/qualityhealth/rights.htm.*

V. Respect and Nondiscrimination

You have a right to considerate, respectful, and nondiscriminatory care from your doctors, health plan representatives, and other health care providers.

VI. Confidentiality of Health Information

You have the right to talk in confidence with health care providers and to have your health care information protected. You also have the right to review and copy your own medical record and request that your physician amend your record if it is not accurate, relevant, or complete.

VII. Complaints and Appeals

You have the right to a fair, fast, and objective review of any complaint you have against your health plan, doctors, hospitals, or other health care personnel. This includes complaints about waiting times, operating hours, the conduct of health care personnel, and the adequacy of health care facilities.

TWO

Choosing the Surgeon
Who Is Best for You

IN THIS CHAPTER

- What makes a surgeon qualified

- How to find a qualified surgeon

- When you need a second opinion

- Personal factors in choosing a surgeon

If you decide to have an operation, choosing your surgeon is one of the most important decisions you will make. Find a competent physician whose specialty is surgery and who is knowledgeable about your medical problem.

WHAT KIND OF SURGEON SHOULD YOU SEE?

You should look for a surgeon with appropriate training, professional qualifications, and experience.

Training

Your first step should be to find a fully trained surgeon. This is a physician who, after medical school, has gone through years of training in an approved training program (called a residency) to learn the specialized skills of a surgeon.

The number of years of residency varies by specialty. (Surgical specialties that the American College of Surgeons, or ACS, recognizes are listed in Appendix B on pages 111 and 112.) A general surgeon, for instance, must complete at least five years of residency training after finishing medical school. A general surgeon is trained in the diagnosis and management of a broad range of surgical conditions.

Some physicians, after they finish their residency, choose to get further training. Fellowship training increases the knowledge and expertise of the specialists in that particular field. They complete a fellowship program in a "subspecialty," a more specialized area of surgery. For instance, general surgeons may choose to specialize in pediatric surgery, hand surgery, minimally invasive surgery, vascular surgery, or surgical critical care. Doctors who completed a plastic surgery residency may extend their training in facial plastic surgery or another subspecialty of plastic surgery. Orthopedic surgeons may specialize in hand surgery or orthopedic sports medicine, and so on. (See Appendix B for a list of subspecialties.)

Whether you decide to see a surgical subspecialist depends on what type of surgical procedure you need and your own preferences. For instance, some general surgeons very competently perform colon surgery, but you may be referred instead to a colon and rectal surgeon who does only that type of work.

Qualifications

A surgeon's training is not the only important credential. The ACS recommends that you look for a surgeon with the following professional qualifications:

Board certification. A good indication of a surgeon's competence is certification by a surgical board that is approved by the American Board of Medical Specialties (ABMS). The ABMS is a not-for-profit organization made up of 24 medical specialty boards that oversee physician certification.

For physicians to become board certified in a surgical specialty, they must complete the years of residency training that their specialty requires. They then must demonstrate their knowledge by passing rigorous exams. It is important that you choose a surgeon who is certified by an ABMS-approved surgical board or by a comparable accrediting agency for osteopathic surgeons.

Practice in an accredited health care facility. Make sure your surgeon has staff privileges to perform surgical procedures at a hospital or in an ambulatory surgery center. Having hospital privileges is important even if the physician is performing your operation in his or her office. Staff privileges show that a hospital review committee has approved the surgeon's qualifications and competency.

It is a good idea to make sure that The Joint Commission or the American Osteopathic Association's Healthcare Facilities Accreditation Program accredited the hospital where your operation will take place. Accreditation means that the health care facility has met high performance and safety standards.

An accreditation option is also available for ambulatory surgical centers. If your operation will take place in this type of facility, you can check to see if the center is accredited by a nationally recognized organization. Accrediting bodies include The Joint Commission, the American Osteopathic Association, the Accreditation Association for Ambulatory Health Care, and the American Association for Accreditation of Ambulatory Surgical Facilities.

When a surgical facility has voluntarily sought accreditation, it is a good sign that it is committed to providing the best possible care for its patients.

Another thing to check is the facility's safety and quality improvement records. To find out if the surgical facility you are considering is accredited by The Joint Commission and to see its quality performance report, visit the commission's Web site at *www.qualitycheck.org.* You can search the site by name of the facility or by state or ZIP code. The American Osteopathic Association also has an online listing of health facilities it accredits. Go to *www.osteopathic.org* and click on Local & Community Resources and then Accredited Health Facilities.

If you need an operation because you have just been diagnosed with cancer, you may want to find an approved cancer program near you. Cancer treatment centers that receive approval by the Commission on Cancer of the American College of Surgeons meet high standards for the quality of care they provide to their patients with cancer. Visit *http:// www.facs.org/cancerprogram/howto.hmtl* to find a center near you.

Fellowship in the American College of Surgeons. A good thing to look for is whether a surgeon is a Fellow of the American College of Surgeons. ACS Fellows have had their education, training, professional qualifications such as board certification, surgical competence, and ethical conduct evaluated and have been found to be consistent with the high standards set by the College.

Not all surgeons are accepted into Fellowship in the College. And some surgeons may choose not to become Fellows.

The letters "FACS" after a surgeon's name indicate that he or she is a Fellow of the American College of Surgeons. These letters show that the surgeon:

• Has volunteered to have peers evaluate his or her credentials and performance

• Is competent to perform surgery

• Has pledged to place the interests of her patients above her own

• Has pledged to follow the ACS Code of Professional Conduct (see pages 20-22 at the end of this chapter)

Verification of credentials. Now that you know what qualifications to look for in selecting a surgeon, how do you check on them? In most cases, surgeons who are board certified and/or Fellows of the ACS will have certificates attesting to these credentials on display in their offices. If not, ask the surgeon or surgeon's office staff to show you these credentials.

There is also a reference book—*The Official ABMS Directory of Board Certified Medical Specialists*—that lists all physicians and surgeons who hold certification from ABMS-approved medical specialty boards. This publication contains brief information about each surgeon's medical education and training. You can find this book in many libraries or through state and county medical associations.

Also, the ABMS Web site (*www.abms.org*) offers "Who's Certified." Through this online service, you can search for a surgeon's board certification status. Or get this information by calling toll-free at 866-ASK-ABMS (275-2267).

You can verify that a surgeon is a Fellow of the ACS by visiting its Web site at *www.facs.org* and clicking on the "Public Information" link at the top of the page. You can also call the College at 312-202-5391.

Experience

Some surgeons specialize in certain surgical procedures. They therefore may have more experience performing these operations. For instance, if you need a hip replacement, you probably would prefer to go to an orthopedic surgeon who mostly performs joint replacements, not one who does hand surgery.

Here's how to learn about a surgeon's experience with the procedure you are considering having. Ask if the surgeon does this operation regularly. However, don't base your decision to use this surgeon only on the volume of operations the surgeon performs. Some procedures are not done very frequently.

Of course, it's not just a surgeon's experience with a procedure that counts. The surgeon's results matter, too. The ACS encourages its members to provide information on their outcomes for their patients. If your surgeon does not give you this information, ask what type of result you can expect after the operation.

You may even want to ask a surgeon to allow you to talk to some of his of her patients. By law, the physician's office must get permission from the patients before releasing their information to you. If a surgeon does not wish to give you patient names, it does not necessarily mean the doctor does not have any patient success stories. The surgeon may not have the time to track down patients and get their consent. But it can't hurt to ask!

These questions also appear at the end of this chapter, under "What to Ask the Surgeon."

HOW CAN YOU FIND A QUALIFIED SURGEON?

The best starting place to find a qualified surgeon is to ask for a referral from the doctor who is treating your medical problem or wants you to talk to a surgeon. If you are a member of a managed care plan and you don't want out-of-pocket costs, make sure that the surgeon your doctor refers you to is in your health plan.

If the doctor cannot recommend a specific surgeon, there are a number of other ways you can find a surgeon. A few ideas follow:

- Talk to a friend who had a similar operation. Ask which physician performed his or her procedure and whether your friend was satisfied with the doctor.

- Find a surgeon in your area through the ACS Web site. (Go to *www.facs.org* and click on the "Public Information" link at the top of the home page.) Or call 312-202-5391.

- Medical specialty societies may have a physician referral phone number or physician finder on their Web sites. See Appendix C for a list of surgical specialty organizations and their contact information.

A PATIENT'S PERSPECTIVE

Andrew Morgavan, 55-year-old who had a back operation in 1998

"My spine surgeon gave me my life back after almost 10 years of back pain due to a back injury. I found my surgeon through my pain management specialist. My wife learned on the Internet about a newly approved back procedure, and I asked my pain specialist about it. He said I would be a good candidate. Coincidentally, it was being done by an orthopedic surgeon who had just joined the same practice that my pain specialist was in. This surgeon had done the new procedure in clinical trials at his previous hospital, so he was exactly what I was looking for. The operation was a complete success."

- Many hospitals and health plans have physician referral services or Web-based physician finders. If you have preferences, such as a surgeon's specialty or gender, share them with the referral service.

SHOULD YOU SEEK A SECOND OPINION?

A second opinion is when another doctor gives his or her view about your medical problem's diagnosis and treatment.

There are no rules to tell you when you need a second or third opinion. It's not like selling real estate! Unlike the common advice to get a market analysis from three real estate agents before listing your home for sale, there is no magic number of surgeons to consult before having an operation.

You probably don't need a second opinion if you feel confident that a surgical procedure is the best treatment for your condition and you are happy with the first surgeon you consulted. And if you need emergency surgery, it is unlikely that you will have time for a second opinion.

However, if your operation is not an emergency, you may want to get a second opinion if:

- You have doubts about the diagnosis or whether to have the operation.

- The doctor recommending the operation is not a qualified surgeon.

- You do not feel comfortable with the surgeon.

Another benefit of visiting a second surgeon is you may learn information important to you that the first surgeon did not mention. A surgeon cannot always cover everything in an initial meeting. Or perhaps the second surgeon will know about a new surgical therapy for your medical problem that the first doctor did not.

If you want a second opinion, you can ask the first surgeon to refer you to another surgeon. Most surgeons won't object to you asking for a second opinion. Or you can ask another doctor you trust to recommend a surgeon. You also can turn to one of the other resources listed in the previous section, "How Can You Find a Qualified Surgeon?"

Before your appointment with the second surgeon, ask the first surgeon to send that doctor copies of any medical tests you had. By doing so, you may not need to repeat these tests when you see the new surgeon.

There's one more important thing to keep in mind. A second opinion is not necessarily better than a first opinion. Whether the two physicians whom you consult agree or disagree on your treatment plan, remember that the final decision to have the operation will be yours. If the two opinions differ and you're not sure what to do, you may want to talk more with the first surgeon. Or you may want to see a third surgeon.

Some hospitals offer a multidisciplinary team approach, which may eliminate the need for the patient to seek a second opinion. The team approach is when specialists in different disciplines (areas) of medicine get together, often with the patient, to review test results and determine the best treatment. This collaborative approach was first used for cancer patients, with the tumor board including the surgeon, medical and radiation oncologists, radiologist, and pathologist.

While still frequently used for cancer care, the team approach also may be offered for other medical problems that typically involve treatment by a variety of health care professionals. Such conditions range from diabetes, epilepsy, and nonhealing wounds, to spine pain, arthritis, and complicated intestinal or vascular problems. The patient benefits from the collective knowledge of both surgeons and nonsurgeons. This approach is helpful when a surgical procedure is not the only form of treatment.

Whether or not you choose to get a second opinion, you should make the decision to have an operation only after you have all the facts. So don't hesitate to discuss with the surgeon any questions or concerns that you may have. *Because all surgical procedures do have some risk, deciding if you should have an operation is a major and obviously important process.* By asking a lot of questions, you'll feel comfortable that you made the right choice.

HOW CAN YOU DECIDE IF A SURGEON IS RIGHT FOR YOU?

The surgeon's training and credentials are not the only factors that will help you choose a surgeon. Your feelings matter, too. You need to feel comfortable with your surgeon. If you have a good doctor-patient relationship, you can more easily communicate with each other. Having good rapport with your surgeon will help you feel confident about the treatment that he or she recommends.

At the first meeting with the surgeon, "size up" the doctor. Consider the surgeon's communication skills. You want a doctor who is interested in you and not distracted or rushed. Your surgeon should take enough time with you.

The surgeon should be willing to answer your questions and should do so in a way you can understand. Sometimes you may have more questions than the surgeon has time for that day. Ask if you can call the surgeon, e-mail your remaining questions, or return for another visit.

Pay attention to the way the surgeon addresses your concerns. The doctor should calm your fears and hesitations about the operation, rather than ignoring them or, even worse, making light of them. Does the surgeon understand why something is important to you? The surgeon should also treat the members of your family the same way you are treated. A good doctor understands the importance of making sure they are as comfortable with this situation as you are.

Professionalism is important also. The surgeon should speak, act, and dress appropriately. He or she should have a positive attitude.

INSIDER'S TIP

Before my recent gallbladder operation, I frequently communicated with my surgeon by e-mail, which worked well for both of us. The fact that he took time to answer my questions about the procedure helped me build a trusting relationship with him. You should work out a means of communication with your surgeon that suits your preferences and the surgeon's schedule, whether that is by phone, fax, e-mail, or in person.

The surgeon's communication skills, ease of contact, professionalism, and staff are all important factors in deciding whether a surgeon is right for you. But the bottom line is: Would you trust your life to this surgeon?

You also should be happy with the surgeon's staff. Are the staff members friendly, respectful, and responsive to your needs? Do they treat your family members with the same courtesy they give you?

A nurse may be the person you see for your first appointment at the surgeon's office. If so, feel free to ask to meet briefly with the surgeon at this time.

Note that a surgeon's age should not be a factor in making your decision. There are no age limits on practicing surgery. The ACS believes that a surgeon's age is not important if the surgeon has current and adequate experience with the surgical procedure and has good results.

DECIDING WHAT'S IMPORTANT TO YOU

The questions that conclude this chapter and those that follow are suggestions for what to ask your surgeon. Most surgeons are excellent in all respects, and the standards for surgery are extremely high in the United States. I suggest these questions because I want to arm you with information you can use to find and access the best doctors in our amazingly good health care system.

You don't need to ask all of the questions on the list if you feel some don't pertain to you or are not useful. As you read the list at the end of each chapter, you may want to highlight the questions you plan to ask your surgeon. Take the list with you to your appointment. Tell your surgeon at the beginning of your visit that you will have questions and ask when the best time to ask them is.

Be respectful, not confrontational, when you ask the surgeon questions. Say that you want to know as much as possible to help you make the right decisions. If you don't feel comfortable asking all the questions you have, bring a trusted family member or friend with you who can help get the information you need.

Code of Professional Conduct for ACS Fellows*

As Fellows of the American College of Surgeons, we treasure the trust that our patients have placed in us, because trust is integral to the practice of surgery. During the continuum of pre-, intra-, and postoperative care, we accept responsibilities to:

- Serve as effective advocates of our patients' needs

- Disclose therapeutic options, including their risks and benefits

- Disclose and resolve any conflict of interest that might influence decisions regarding care

- Be sensitive and respectful of patients, understanding their vulnerability during the perioperative period

- Fully disclose adverse events and medical errors

- Acknowledge patients' psychological, social, cultural, and spiritual needs

- Encompass within our surgical care the special needs of terminally ill patients

- Acknowledge and support the needs of patients' families

- Respect the knowledge, dignity, and perspective of other health care professionals

Our profession is also accountable to our communities and to society. In return for their trust, as Fellows of the American College of Surgeons, we accept responsibilities to:

- Provide the highest quality surgical care

- Abide by the values of honesty, confidentiality, and altruism

- Participate in lifelong learning

- Maintain competence throughout our surgical careers

- Participate in self-regulation by setting, maintaining, and enforcing practice standards

- Improve care by evaluating its processes and outcomes

- Inform the public about subjects within our expertise

- Advocate strategies to improve individual and public health by communicating with government, health care organizations, and industry

- Work with society to establish just, effective, and efficient distribution of health care resources

- Provide necessary surgical care without regard to gender, race, disability, religion, social status, or ability to pay

- Participate in educational programs addressing professionalism

---

*Approved by the American College of Surgeons (ACS) Board of Regents, June 2003.

What to Ask the Surgeon

About the Surgeon

☐ What kind of surgery were you trained to do?

☐ Are you board certified in the surgical specialty in which you practice?

☐ Do you have staff privileges to perform surgical procedures at an accredited health care facility?

☐ Are you a member of the American College of Surgeons?

☐ Do you have any health problems that would interfere with your ability to do this operation?

☐ Are you a member of my managed care network?

About Results

☐ How many of these operations do you do in a year?

☐ What type of result can I expect based on the results of the operation for other patients of yours?

☐ What is your percentage success rate with this operation? Do you have your outcomes in writing?

☐ What is your safety record regarding complications?

☐ Can I talk to some of your patients who have had you perform this operation for them?

☐ If I have more questions, what is the best way to contact you?

THREE

What to Ask the Surgeon at the First Meeting

IN THIS CHAPTER

- What you should know to decide whether to have the operation

- How you can improve the odds of having a good surgical result

- What details you should know now about the operation

When you buy a new car, you gather facts about the vehicle you're interested in purchasing. You may read information, ask car salespeople questions, and talk to people who own that model.

When you need an operation, you should go through a similar research process to become informed. Unfortunately, you can't test drive an operation! Consider this chapter, then, to be the manual for your first visit with a surgeon.

During your first meeting with a surgeon, you will decide if the surgeon is right for you, as discussed in Chapter 2. You also will learn to ask whether a certain operation is the best treatment for your medical problem and what the risks and benefits of the procedure are, all of which is the focus of this chapter. You may have specific questions about preparing for the operation, some of which I address in this chapter.

Chapter 4 goes into more detail about preoperative concerns, including anesthesia options. You may want to read it as well before your first visit with the surgeon.

Some hospitals offer surgical patients and their families an information program to help them prepare for an operation. Check with your hospital to see if it has this kind of patient education program.

Your first meeting may be your only visit with the surgeon before you have the operation. It is likely, though, that you will need more than one visit if the operation is not an emergency. For instance, if you schedule your elective operation for weeks or months after your first visit, the surgeon probably will want to see you again right before the operation. This meeting will give you a chance to ask last-minute questions and for the surgeon to examine you and make sure you are healthy enough for the operation.

Remember, if you don't understand the surgeon's answers to your questions, keep asking until you do understand. It is helpful to bring a family member or friend with you to your appointment. That person may think to ask questions that you forgot and will help you remember more of what the surgeon says.

DO YOU REALLY NEED THE OPERATION?

A surgical procedure is generally not the first treatment for a health problem. It usually is done after other treatments have been exhausted. Before you choose to have an operation, you should be convinced that your medical problem will not get better on its own or with nonsurgical treatment.

During your initial visit, ask the surgeon, Why do I need an operation? What will happen if I don't have the operation now? Are there medical treatments or lifestyle changes that can help me avoid or postpone an operation?

If you are unclear about exactly what is wrong with you or how the operation will help your problem, now is the time to ask!

Should your surgeon recommend that you have an operation right away, make sure you understand why. Consider asking the doctor who sent you to the surgeon if your condition is urgent. If you don't feel com-

A PATIENT'S PERSPECTIVE

Debbie Ryan, 53-year-old who had cancer of the pancreas surgically removed in 2000

"I was feeling sick and went to a digestive disease specialist. Tests showed a mass on a pancreatic duct, and a biopsy came back negative [normal]. But my surgeon thought it might be cancer, and he wanted to operate right away. I didn't think it was cancer and was hesitant to have an operation. He didn't say, 'You're going to do this.' He gave me time to decide what I wanted to do. He allowed me to find my own way. I had to know the surgeon would listen to what I wanted. Otherwise he wouldn't be the surgeon for me. His concern led me to schedule an operation two days later. When I woke up from the operation, I found out the mass was malignant, and he had removed the cancer. I also had chemo and radiation therapy. I've been cancer free for six years."

fortable with the urgency, consider getting a second opinion. If your condition is not life-threatening, take a little time to decide whether to have the operation.

WHAT ARE THE TREATMENT OPTIONS?

Some medical problems have just a few treatment options. For instance, an operation is the only treatment for acute, ruptured appendicitis. For other diseases, such as prostate or breast cancer, there are many different treatment options or ways to perform the operation. Some surgical procedures use a surgical device, such as a spinal fusion device in spine surgery or an intraocular lens in cataract surgery. So you may have various options for the type of device used.

Your surgeon will discuss the medical and surgical options you have. The more options you are aware of, the better informed the decision you will make.

You also may want to research your treatment options before you meet with the surgeon. Read patient education materials and books on your condition, visit medical Web sites, and so on. The American College of Surgeons, for instance, has a patient education Web site (*www.facs.org/patienteducation/index.html*). It provides patients with the most current information about surgical procedures, diseases, tests, medications, and pain management.

Often an operation is a treatment option for cancer. The American Cancer Society Web site (*www.cancer.org*) provides treatment option decision tools based on your type of tumor and its stage.

Even if you have already decided on a treatment approach based on your research, have an open mind when you speak with the surgeon. Remember that the surgeon takes into consideration your overall health status and knows the specific details of your condition. Your surgeon will work with you to weigh the pros and cons of each surgical approach, helping you to decide on the best option considering your health and lifestyle. Find out which surgical procedure the doctor recommends, and why. Ask the surgeon, "Would you recommend this operation if I were your relative or if you were the patient?"

While discussing treatment options, if your surgeon does not mention a new or evolving treatment that you are aware of, ask about his or her experience with it and opinion about it. If the surgeon recommends a traditional approach instead of the new treatment, ask why. When the answer is not what you want to hear, get a second opinion. But remember, new is not always better, and not every treatment is right for every patient.

Some new treatments are considered experimental, because doctors are still studying them to learn if they are safe and effective. Clinical trials—research studies that test a new treatment in people—sometimes are the only way to get treatment with certain new surgical devices or drugs in the United States. Thus, participation in a clinical trial may offer a promising therapy for someone whose medical problem does not have an easy solution or that has a poor prognosis. If you have not had success with standard treatments for your condition, ask your surgeon if there are any ongoing clinical trials for patients with your problem. This is an option primarily for problems related to cancer. Two Web sites that are good resources on clinical trials are one provided by the American College of Surgeons Oncology Group at *www.acosog.org,* and another from the US National Institutes of Health at *http://clinicaltrials.gov.*

WHAT ARE THE RISKS AND BENEFITS?

Every surgical procedure poses some risk for the patient. Risks include possible side effects, such as pain or swelling around the incision site, and potential complications during or after the operation—for example, excessive bleeding or infection. You must weigh the risks against the expected benefits.

For some people, having an operation is too risky. Some reasons may be:

• Poor health (lung disease, heart problems, liver disease, and so on)

• Advanced age along with poor health

• A tumor that lies too close to a vital organ or blood vessel and is deemed inoperable

If you have any other health problems, be sure to tell your surgeon. It may make a difference in what type of operation or anesthesia you have, or how you are monitored.

For many people the benefits of having an operation outweigh the risks. For instance, one of the risks of treatment of prostate cancer is urinary incontinence (inability to control one's bladder), yet treatment has the benefit of likely curing the cancer.

Ask your surgeon what the chance of complications is. If a certain risk is higher than you feel comfortable with, ask if it can be prevented or minimized and how a complication would be treated if it happens.

WHAT RESULTS CAN YOU EXPECT?

You obviously want to know if the operation will have the result you want: a cure, restored health, relief of your symptoms, a return to function, and so forth. Ask, too, about the effect of the operation on your quality of life. Will it alter your lifestyle? Will you need continuing treatment to counter any adverse effects of the operation if they occur?

You'll also want to know the average success rate of the operation. Don't forget to ask if the surgeon does this particular operation regularly and how many does he or she perform during a year's time? What are that surgeon's typical results for patients who have this surgical procedure? What percentage of the surgeon's patients have serious complications?

Understand, however, that it is impossible for a surgeon to exactly predict results. No doctor can, or should, guarantee outcomes. Each operation is different, depending on the individual condition and the physical response of each patient. Nonetheless, your surgeon will be able to give you a good idea of what to expect.

HOW LONG WILL IT TAKE YOU TO RECOVER?

Of course, you will want to know how long to expect before you can return to work, school, or other regular activities. Your surgeon can give you an estimate, but again, your recovery may be shorter or longer than average.

WHAT CAN YOU DO TO IMPROVE CHANCES OF A GOOD OUTCOME?

As an active participant in the surgical process, you can take steps even before the operation to help increase the likelihood that you'll have a good result. I've already mentioned one way: by becoming informed about your treatment options and their risks versus benefits.

In addition, be honest when the surgeon takes your health history. Tell the doctor if you abuse drugs or alcohol. Regular use of certain drugs, such as anabolic steroids or opiate painkillers, can increase the risks during anesthesia. And studies have shown that heavy drinking increases the risk of postoperative problems.

Also, you should carefully follow your surgeon's preoperative instructions so that you will have the best chance of a good outcome.

Here's another way to up the odds of surgical success: improve your general health before the operation.

Under your doctor's supervision, start an exercise program or work out more regularly. If you're overweight or underweight, which can increase your surgical risks, try to reach a healthier weight.

If you smoke, stop smoking—at least a few weeks before the operation, if not for good. Smoking cigarettes delays healing after an operation and increases the risk of infection.

HOW WILL THE OPERATION BE PERFORMED?

The surgeon will explain how he or she will do the operation and what kind of anesthesia you will receive. (For more information about anesthesia options, see Chapter 4.)

Some operations are done only with the traditional open technique, in which the surgeon makes a cut in your body. Increasingly more operations involve minimally invasive techniques using several tiny incisions. Into one of these small holes, the surgeon inserts a small lighted viewing tube similar to a telescope. A miniature TV camera is at the end of the scope, and it magnifies images onto a monitor in the operating room (OR). The surgeon then inserts surgical instruments into the other openings.

This type of operation is called laparoscopy for abdominal procedures, thoracoscopy in the chest, arthroscopy in the joints, and other names depending on the site.

Advantages of minimally invasive surgery include less bleeding and pain, faster healing and return to normal activities, and fewer complications, such as infection. It may also reduce the need for an overnight stay in the hospital.

Almost any invasive surgical procedure has a less invasive alternative. Examples include:

- Gallbladder removal

- Removal of the appendix

- Hernia repair

- Removal of uterine fibroid tumors

- Sinus operation

- Cardiovascular procedures, such as angioplasty and stent placement

- Weight reduction (bariatric) surgical procedure

- Tumor removal

Small-incision surgery is not right for everyone. Ask your surgeon if your operation can be done using small incisions and if you are a candidate for this approach. If so, ask how large the incisions will be and where on your body.

Find out if there is a chance that the surgeon will need to convert the operation to an open, or traditional, approach, so you can be prepared for that possibility. This change may occur if the procedure turns out to be more complex than expected.

WHO ELSE IS ON THE SURGICAL TEAM?

The surgeon is the leader of the surgical team, but there are many other team members. They include the anesthesia professional, OR nurses, and OR technicians. You may want to ask if the surgeon has worked with this team before.

It is also appropriate to ask if there will be another surgeon assisting in the operation. If you are having the operation at a teaching hospital, a resident (surgeon in training) may perform parts of the procedure under the surgeon's close supervision.

IN WHAT FACILITY WILL THE OPERATION BE PERFORMED?

The surgeon may perform the operation in the hospital, in an ambulatory surgery center, or in his or her office. Ask your surgeon where the operation will be done and if this is the type of place where your operation is typically done. If not, ask why the surgeon recommends a different setting.

Today most operations can be done in your community. You don't automatically need to go to a university teaching hospital, even if you have a complex medical problem or need a major operation. Whichever surgical facility you choose, make sure that:

- The surgical facility is accredited (see Chapter 2) as well as properly staffed and equipped (see Chapter 4).

- The surgical team has experience doing the procedure you need and does it on a regular basis.

- The surgeon or the facility has data on outcomes for the specific procedure.

- The facility has a good safety record (*see www.qualitycheck.org*).

If you are not satisfied that your community hospital or surgical center meets these criteria, you may want to consult a surgeon at a major academic medical center.

WHICH TESTS WILL YOU NEED BEFORE THE OPERATION?

Sometimes a surgeon will order medical tests, such as blood work or imaging studies. Your doctor may need to perform tests right away or days before the operation to:

- Confirm your diagnosis or the severity of the problem

- Verify that you need this operation or determine the best surgical approach

- Pinpoint the site that needs surgical intervention and determine that the procedure can be safely and effectively done

- Determine if you are healthy enough to safely undergo the operation

Preoperative tests make sure you are not anemic (have iron-deficient blood) and that your kidneys and liver are functioning properly. Other tests may check for heart or lung problems. If the doctor suspects cancer, a biopsy (see Glossary) may be performed to test for malignant cells.

If there is a chance that you will need a blood transfusion during a major operation, a sample of your blood will be taken to find out what blood type you are. You can ask about donating your own blood in advance of the operation if it's possible you will need a transfusion. (For more information, see Chapter 4.)

WHAT DOES "INFORMED CONSENT" MEAN?

Before having your operation, you will be asked to give your written permission for the operation. You will be asked to read a consent form, which indicates that you understand the nature of the surgical procedure to be performed. This process is called "informed consent."

It may appear to be a formality, but, in fact, the informed consent process should be taken very seriously. Frankly discuss with your surgeon any questions or concerns that you have now so that you will be ready to sign the form later (usually right before the operation). Remember, the operation is being performed on you, and you should seek any information you need to improve your understanding. Your doctor should be willing to take whatever time you need to make sure you are fully informed.

Children do not sign an informed consent form. Their adult parent or guardian does. However, children over age 13 are usually asked to give consent for the procedure, even though their parents sign the legal document.

The American College of Surgeons endorses the principle of informed consent. Its *Statements on Principles* say, in part, "Patients should understand the indications for the operation, the risk involved, and the result that it is hoped to attain."

The questions at the end of this chapter provide a checklist for you to make sure the surgeon has covered all of this information.

WILL YOU NEED TO MAKE ARRANGEMENTS FOR AFTER THE OPERATION?

Find out if you will require any special care after your operation. Will you need to stay in an extended-care facility after you leave the hospital? Arrange for home health care? Get physical therapy or other rehab? Finding out now will give you time to prepare.

WILL THE SURGEON BE AVAILABLE AFTER THE OPERATION?

If you require a hospital stay, ask: Will you or an equally qualified surgeon in your practice visit me in the hospital after my operation? Sometimes surgeons have to be away because they have to work at another hospital, attend a clinical meeting, or even take vacation time! When that happens, another surgeon in the practice should be available to help with your care. Your surgeon or a designated physician should at least be available by phone if your nurse needs to get an order for a test or a change in prescription. It is your surgeon's job to manage your postoperative care.

Ask if other physicians will be involved in your care while you're in the hospital. For instance, you may see a hospitalist, a doctor who specializes in hospital care and stays in close communication with your surgeon and primary care doctor. Or if you have a heart problem, you may need to see a cardiologist.

You will need to ask your primary care physician if he or she will visit you in the hospital. Many do not, because they focus on office-based care.

Even if you are having an outpatient operation, you may have problems or questions when you get home. Make sure your surgeon plans to be available, even on weekends and holidays.

INSIDER'S TIP

Be aware that if you schedule your operation right before a holiday, the hospital may be short-staffed during the holiday. Your surgeon may even go on vacation after performing your operation! Ask about the surgeon's availability at that time.

If you will be at a teaching hospital, bear in mind that a new group of first-year house staff (physicians in training) arrives July 1, and the senior house staff graduates and leaves. If you are planning on having an operation at an academic medical center, you may want to ask your surgeon if it is an appropriate time to schedule the procedure.

When you schedule your operation, ask to be the surgeon's first case of the day to avoid having your procedure delayed.

What to Ask the Surgeon

☐ Why do I need an operation?

☐ What are the treatment options?

☐ Which treatment approach do you recommend?

☐ What are the risks and benefits?

☐ What results can I expect?

☐ Do you perform this operation regularly? What are your results?

☐ Will I need a blood transfusion?

☐ Will any transplanted tissue, grafts, implanted devices, plates, or screws be used? What do I need to know about them?

☐ How long will it take me to recover?

☐ What can I do to improve my chances of a good outcome?

☐ How will you perform the operation?

☐ Who else is on the surgical team?

☐ In what facility will you do the operation?

☐ What kind of tests will I need before the operation?

☐ Will I need to make advance arrangements for care or therapy after the operation?

☐ Will you visit me in the hospital after my operation?

☐ How much will the operation cost, how will the costs be billed, and what kind of insurance coverage do you accept?

FOUR

Preparing for the Operation

IN THIS CHAPTER

- Safety of the surgical facility

- Anesthesia options

- Typical preoperative instructions

- Importance of preparing physically and emotionally for the operation

- Financial and insurance considerations

- What to ask the surgeon

You've made the decision to have an operation, you've picked the surgeon, and you've met with that physician at least once. Now you'll want specifics on what you need to do to be ready for the surgical procedure.

Being prepared is being smart. That's why this chapter covers the preparations that many people don't want to think about, such as living wills and financial costs. These are not your top concerns, obviously, but they are important.

Typically, the surgeon goes over preoperative details during a visit before the operation. The surgeon's office or the surgical facility may have this information in writing. In that case, you'll want to read that material as well as this chapter.

You can expect a call from an admitting nurse at the surgical facility a day or two before the procedure. The nurse will give you specific information about your operation.

Preoperative information varies depending on the procedure and the patient. It is important to follow your doctor's and surgical facility's instructions, which are specific to your procedure. Use this chapter as a general guide for what to expect and what to ask at your "preop" visit.

IS THE SURGICAL FACILITY PROPERLY STAFFED AND EQUIPPED?

You've already made sure that the surgical facility is accredited (Chapter 2). There are other details you should find out to help ensure your safety.

Many surgical procedures now take place in outpatient surgical centers and doctors' offices, rather than a hospital operating room. If the operation will occur at a facility other than a hospital, find out what safety measures are in place in case there are complications and you need to be transferred to the hospital. The surgeon should have either admitting privileges to a nearby hospital or an emergency transfer arrangement there.

You also may want to ask if the surgeon has staff privileges to perform the procedure at the hospital if necessary. Having staff privileges shows that a hospital review committee has approved the surgeon's qualifications and competency.

Also, ask whether the surgical center or doctor's office has defibrillators and other life-saving equipment as well as rescue drugs in case of an anesthesia overdose. If you are not comfortable with the reply, ask the surgeon to perform the procedure at a hospital that does have the proper rescue equipment.

To make sure the facility has the proper staff for administering anesthesia, see the "Anesthesia Providers" section.

INSIDER'S TIP

Throughout the United States, there is a nursing shortage. If you plan a hospital stay, find out what the patient-to-nurse ratio is. Ask your surgeon or a nurse manager at the hospital. Studies have shown that patient safety suffers when nursing staffing is low, because nurses have too many patients to take care of adequately. Nurse ratios typically depend on multiple factors, including the number of patients in the unit, the patients' care needs (postoperative recovery, intensive care, general inpatient, and so on), and the nurses' skill level and experience.

Ask your surgeon if the ratio of nurses to patients is appropriate and adequate for the type of procedure you are having and for your needs. The ratio should be adequate, not just during the day but also at night.

WHAT ARE YOUR OPTIONS FOR ANESTHESIA?

Anesthesia, the medically induced loss of sensitivity to pain, is a major part of your operation. Have your surgeon explain the types of anesthesia available to you as well as their benefits and risks.

Types of Anesthesia

The type of anesthesia you will receive depends on the nature of your surgical procedure, your health, and your age. Your anesthesia provider also will consider your personal preferences if possible. You will receive one or more of four types of anesthesia.

- *General anesthesia:* You will be unconscious (asleep) during the procedure. Major operations usually are performed this way. You will get the anesthetic medicine through an intravenous (IV) line hooked up to your arm or hand, or as a gas through an anesthesia mask. Sometimes the anesthesiologist may give you the anesthesia through a temporary breathing tube placed through your mouth and into your

windpipe after you are asleep. Beforehand, you may receive sedatives. These medications make you calm and drowsy, in preparation
for general anesthesia.

- *Regional anesthesia:* You will receive an injection (shot) of a numbing local anesthetic into the nerves supplying the area to be operated
on. This type of anesthesia is used when a large area needs numbing,
such as an arm or leg or the lower half of your body. You also may
receive sedatives, which may dim your memory of the procedure.

- *Local anesthesia:* The doctor numbs a small area of skin near the place
where the incision will be made, so that a painless cut can be made.
A local anesthetic can be given as a shot or applied to the skin as an
ointment or spray. If the medicine is applied to the skin, your doctor
may call it a topical anesthetic. Local anesthesia often is used for
minor outpatient procedures and does not require an anesthesia professional (see "Anesthesia Providers" in the next section for a defini-
tion). You remain fully alert during the procedure.

- *Conscious sedation:* Formerly called twilight anesthesia, this technique
uses sedatives to lower your level of consciousness without putting
you into a deep sleep, as in general anesthesia. These medications
cause temporary forgetfulness, so you may not remember the procedure. Depending on the level of sedation, you may be awake and able
to talk to the surgeon or respond physically to the surgical team's questions or requests. You will receive pain medicine, usually through an
IV. You also may get a local or regional anesthetic.

With conscious sedation, it is sometimes possible for the patient to
reach a deeper level of sedation than intended. For this reason, guidelines
state that all patients should be monitored during conscious sedation,
including their blood pressure and pulse. In addition, a monitor will be
placed on your finger to determine oxygen saturation and to make sure
that your breathing is adequate. It is advisable that an anesthesia professional or other qualified health care provider be dedicated to monitoring
a patient receiving conscious sedation. The person who will monitor your

condition during the procedure should have training in monitoring breathing and heart function and should be trained to take immediate corrective action if sedation becomes too deep. This professional should stay with you during the entire procedure.

Anesthesia Providers

Unless your surgical procedure requires only local anesthesia, you should expect that an anesthesia professional will assist your surgeon. This person will be a physician (anesthesiologist) or nurse (nurse anesthetist) who has received special training in anesthesia and is licensed to administer anesthesia. In some states, other persons, such as dental hygienists, are licensed to give conscious sedation.

If your surgeon will be the one administering anesthesia or conscious sedation, make sure that he or she is trained in anesthesia or conscious sedation as well as safety practices such as resuscitation. Ask if there will be a qualified person other than your surgeon who will continuously monitor your vital signs.

Usually you won't meet the anesthesia provider until right before your operation. At some surgical facilities, an anesthesia professional calls the patient the day before the procedure to explain the anesthesia technique and special requirements. If you have concerns or questions about the anesthesia, ask to speak with an anesthesia professional in advance or arrange a meeting.

What to Tell the Anesthesia Provider

Tell the anesthesia provider if you:

- Have had problems with anesthesia in the past

- Have drug or food allergies or other health problems

- Are taking medications or vitamins

- Have dentures, crowns, or loose teeth

- Have ongoing major health problems such as seizures or heart or lung disease

• Have a recent-onset illness that might affect the operation, such as a cold or flu, skin infection, or severe diarrhea

Unfortunately, vomiting is one of the potential side effects of anesthesia. Tell the anesthesia provider if you threw up from anesthesia in a past operation. Newer medicines are available that may prevent vomiting. You also can ask to receive antinausea drugs, which may help.

Will I Wake Up During the Operation?

Some patients fear that they will wake up while they are on the operating table. Such unexpected awakening during general anesthesia is called surgical (or intraoperative) awareness. In most cases of surgical awareness, the patient does not feel pain, because the painkillers continue to work.

Let me reassure you that this problem is rare. It happens in less than 0.1 or 0.2 percent of operations, according to a 2006 report by the American Society of Anesthesiologists. And recent advances may make this problem even rarer. There are efforts to monitor a patient's brain activity in an attempt to better determine the proper anesthetic dose.

WHEN SHOULD YOU STOP EATING BEFORE THE OPERATION?

Your stomach needs to be empty for your operation. An empty stomach decreases the risks of vomiting and aspiration (getting food particles into your lungs), which can lead to pneumonia.

You must stop eating and drinking at least four hours before the operation. This may vary depending on the time scheduled for your procedure. Your surgeon will tell you what applies to you. Sometimes you will not know the exact time of the surgical procedure until the day before the operation.

If you are told to fast (stop eating), you also must not chew gum or suck on candy, mints, or cough drops.

For a procedure needing just local anesthesia, you probably will not need to fast.

WHAT MEDICATIONS CAN YOU TAKE BEFORE THE OPERATION?

Come to your surgeon with a list of all the medications you take (both prescription and over-the-counter). Include vitamins and herbal supplements on this list. Some supplements and herbs may cause negative effects when combined with general anesthesia.

Ask your doctor or nurse which of your usual drugs you can and cannot take the day of the operation.

Some medicines need to be stopped before an operation. For instance, you should stop taking Plavix®, aspirin, and anti-inflammatory drugs such as ibuprofen three days or more before a surgical procedure. (Some doctors recommend stopping aspirin and aspirin-like drugs two weeks before an operation, so check with your surgeon.) These drugs interfere with blood clotting and can cause excessive bleeding during the procedure. If you take a blood thinner such as Plavix®, aspirin, warfarin, or heparin, tell your surgeon, who may ask you to stop taking it. After you stop taking a blood thinner, your doctor may check your blood for proper clotting.

You also may need to discontinue taking vitamins E and C, certain herbal supplements, and weight-loss medications. Always ask your health care professional before stopping a medication.

Your surgeon may instruct you to continue taking some medications, such as heart medicine, diabetes medicine, steroids, or blood pressure medicine. He or she may also ask you to take antibiotics before and after the operation to help prevent you from developing an infection. On the day of the operation, take any required drugs with a sip of water.

WHAT KIND OF CLOTHING SHOULD YOU WEAR?

Wear comfortable, loose clothing on the day of your operation. It should be easy to remove and fold.

ARE THERE ANY OTHER PREOPERATIVE INSTRUCTIONS?

Don't wear makeup, and remove jewelry. Leave jewelry and other valuables at home. If you wear nail polish, you will need to remove it. The surgical team must see the natural color of your fingernails to check your circulation. If you wear artificial nails, ask if you need to remove them.

Your surgeon will give you any other instructions you need to follow. For instance, some bowel operations need special preparation to empty the bowel.

Your doctor or anesthesia provider may tell you not to drink alcohol before the operation.

If you smoke, your surgeon may recommend that you not smoke before the operation. You should follow this advice, even though it may be difficult. A reduction in smoking lowers the risk of respiratory problems, such as pneumonia, after a surgical procedure. Also, healing will improve if you don't smoke.

When you have medical problems besides the one you are having surgical treatment for, you may need to get clearance from your primary care physician to have the operation.

Commonly, patients need preop tests, such as blood work or a urine test, to make sure they are healthy enough to undergo the operation. Your surgeon will let you know if you need tests before the operation.

If you become ill right before your operation, such as from a cold, fever, infection, or bleeding disorder, call your surgeon. You may have to postpone the surgical procedure until you are well.

HOW LONG WILL YOU HAVE TO STAY IN THE HOSPITAL OR SURGICAL CENTER?

When you can go home after an operation will depend on the type of procedure you have and the anesthesia that is used. Your length of stay at the surgical facility will vary from hours for an outpatient procedure to overnight or longer for an inpatient operation. Ask your surgeon for an estimate of when you can expect to return home.

Occasionally after an outpatient operation, you may need to stay overnight. If your operation will take place in a freestanding surgical center, ask your surgeon which hospital you will go to if you need an overnight stay. Most outpatient surgical centers do not have overnight facilities.

If you want a private room in the hospital, tell your surgeon or the hospital admitting staff.

WILL YOU NEED SOMEONE TO DRIVE YOU HOME?

Most often you will need a ride home from the surgical facility. You will not be allowed to drive yourself if you have had sedation or anesthesia. So you can plan ahead, ask if you need to arrange for a ride home.

IS IT POSSIBLE YOU'LL NEED BLOOD TRANSFUSIONS?

Some patients believe that having an operation means they will need a blood transfusion. This is not so. Most planned surgical procedures do not cause enough blood loss to result in the need for a blood transfusion. A physician will transfuse a patient only when necessary.

Sometimes, however, a surgeon can expect the amount of blood lost during an operation to be large enough to require a transfusion. Some types of operations that commonly cause large blood loss are:

- Heart or chest surgical procedures

- Vascular operations

- Hip or knee replacement

- Major spine surgical procedures

- Radical prostatectomy (surgical removal of the entire prostate)

- Liver resection

Ask your surgeon if the need for a blood transfusion is likely with your operation. If so, know that our nation's blood supply undergoes careful routine medical testing to screen for infectious diseases, such as AIDS and viral hepatitis (a liver disease). These tests are highly accurate.

Donating Your Own Blood

If there's a good chance you'll need a transfusion and you would prefer to use your own blood rather than blood from an anonymous donor, ask if you can donate your blood ahead of time. This technique is called autologous (aw-tol'-o-gus) donation. Autologous means "related to self." Most doctors recommend that patients undergoing an operation consider autologous donation only when there is a reasonable probability that they will require a blood transfusion.

This type of donation is not appropriate for everyone. The operation must be scheduled at least several weeks in advance. You can't give blood later than 72 hours before the operation, and there must be time between donations of units of blood.

Your body replaces the blood you donated in a matter of weeks. By donating blood for yourself before an operation, you do not increase the risk of bleeding during the procedure.

If you give your own blood and you don't need blood after the operation, it usually cannot be donated to someone else. If blood can be donated, it must be screened for infectious diseases in the same way as for regular donors.

Most patients having an elective operation can donate their own blood. Check with your insurance plan whether it covers the cost.

If you cannot give your own blood (because you are anemic, for example), ask your surgeon about other options for blood transfusion. For instance, you may be able to use a designated donor, such as a friend or relative, who has agreed to donate blood in the event that you need it. The blood donation has to be done several days in advance of your operation.

DO YOU NEED A LIVING WILL?

Every adult should have a living will. If you don't, now is a good time to get one.

A living will is not the same as a will. It is a written record of the health care you would want if you were unable to make medical decisions for yourself because you have a terminal illness or you are permanently unconscious (in a coma). A living will spells out if you want to accept or refuse life support and other care that artificially postpones dying. This legal form allows you to say what measures, if any, you want health care providers to take to try to keep you alive. Life-prolonging treatments include cardiopulmonary resuscitation (CPR), a respirator, and tube feeding. If you refuse life-prolonging treatments, you will still receive pain medicine and care to keep you comfortable.

You should appoint someone to follow the directions in your living will. You can make this appointment by using a written form called a "Durable Power of Attorney for Health Care" or a "Medical Durable Power of Attorney." This statement allows you to pick someone who will make decisions about your medical treatment in the event that you cannot. This person is called a health care agent, proxy, surrogate, or guardian, depending on the state where you live.

A living will and power of attorney are called advance directives.

Why Advance Directives Are Important

If you do not have a health care power of attorney, and you cannot make your own decisions, your family may not know what treatment you would want. So you should have both a medical power of attorney and a living will. It is better to put them in writing because not all states accept oral advance directives as being legal. Also, be sure to check to see if living wills and power of attorney are considered to be advanced directives in the state where you live.

Federal law (the Patient Self-Determination Act of 1990) requires most hospitals to ask if you have advance directives and to document that fact in your medical record.

Where to Get Advance Directives

Laws concerning advance directives vary by state. To get forms for advance directives that apply in your state, contact your lawyer or hospital patient representative. You also may find these forms on the Internet—for example, through the Web site of your state's attorney's office or your state's department of public health.

Give copies of your advance directives to your surgeon, the surgical facility, your health care power of attorney, and your immediate family.

HOW CAN YOU PREPARE YOURSELF EMOTIONALLY?

It is normal to feel anxious about having a surgical procedure. You should feel free to discuss any concerns or fears you have about the operation with your surgeon. Part of the surgeon's job is to help prepare you physically and psychologically for the operation.

I've already talked about the importance of getting your body in the best shape possible before a surgical procedure. But it is also important to feel comfortable with having an operation. Postoperative outcomes tend to be better for patients who are emotionally and physically ready for a surgical procedure.

Getting information from your surgeon and from this book is a great way to prepare emotionally. Being informed may ease most of your worries. However, if you have remaining concerns, talk to your primary care physician or to patients who have had this operation.

In the days before your operation, you may want to use relaxation techniques. Some relaxation techniques are meditation, prayer, deep breathing, yoga, and massage therapy.

If you are still not emotionally ready to have the surgical procedure and your condition is not an emergency, tell your surgeon you need more time.

A PATIENT'S PERSPECTIVE

Margaret Telow, 46-year-old who had both hips replaced in 2005 because of arthritis

"My orthopedic surgeon gave me a lot of time to talk about my fears. I asked him about rumors I had heard. Is it true that after hip replacement I'll never be able to cross my legs again? He told me that was not true, and I laughed at myself. I was also afraid of having two operations and not having control of my family. I have a handicapped son who needs my care. I asked if I could have both hips replaced at one time: what the benefits were, whether the recovery was longer or the risks were greater. I decided to have a double hip replacement.

Before the operation, the pain was so bad, I couldn't walk to my car without crying from the pain. Now the pain is totally gone. I'm happy I had the operation."

WHAT ABOUT MANAGED CARE AND INSURANCE POLICIES?

Your operation may be less worrisome if you find out in advance what it will cost. You should already have made sure that your insurance plan covers your surgeon and the surgical facility. Now discuss with your surgeon his or her fees and those of his assistants.

Many surgeons may volunteer this information. If yours does not, don't hesitate to ask. The American College of Surgeons encourages its members to frankly discuss fees and payment with their patients. Your surgeon may have an employee in his or her business office who can discuss fees and payment policies with you.

Physicians and hospitals bill separately for their services. The hospital will bill for the operating room and hospitalization if needed. For information about hospital charges, contact your hospital's business office. Many states require hospitals to publicly report patient charges. However, some hospitals do not give out this information. Fortunately, the health care system is moving to be more open, or transparent, about costs. There is a growing emphasis for health care providers and facilities to give patients this pricing information, which is called cost transparency.

You also should expect to receive separate bills for the professional services of others involved in your care. These people may include the assisting surgeon, anesthesia provider, pathologists, radiologists, and medical consultants.

Understand the coverage of your medical benefit plan before your hospitalization so that you will know what portion of the costs will be yours (your "out-of-pocket" costs). Your doctor's office staff may be able to help you find out how much your health insurance plan will cover. If not, call your health plan.

If your plan will not pay all of the anticipated surgeon's costs (or if you have a high deductible) and you cannot afford the difference, discuss the situation frankly with your surgeon. See if you can work out a solution that is mutually acceptable.

To make payment arrangements for the hospital share of the costs, speak to the hospital's financial advisor. Or check to see if the hospital has a social worker who can help you find financial assistance if you are eligible.

Finally, some insurance plans require preauthorization (also called precertification) before an operation and hospital stay. It is different from preregistration, which is explained in Chapter 5 and may be an option at your surgical facility. Preauthorization requires a plan member or the doctor in charge of the member's care to notify the insurer, in advance, of plans for major care such as a hospital admission. Find out if you need to get preauthorization, so you won't get any unpleasant surprises after the operation.

What to Ask the Surgeon

☐ Is the surgical facility properly staffed and equipped?

☐ What are my options for anesthesia?

☐ When should I stop eating before the operation?

☐ What medications am I allowed to take before the operation? And which need to be stopped?

☐ What kind of clothing should I wear?

☐ Are there any other special preoperative instructions?

☐ How long will I have to stay in the hospital or surgical center?

☐ Will I need someone to drive me home?

☐ Is it possible I'll need a blood transfusion?

☐ Do I need a living will?

☐ How can I prepare myself emotionally?

☐ What about managed care and insurance policies? What will be my out-of-pocket costs?

FIVE

Having the Operation

IN THIS CHAPTER	

- What to bring to the surgical facility

- How to help make sure you get the right surgical procedure on the correct place on your body

- What happens behind closed doors in the operating room and recovery room

- What you and your family should ask the surgeon

WHAT SHOULD YOU BRING TO THE SURGICAL FACILITY?

Here is a list of what to bring with you to the surgical facility on the day of the operation:

- Identification (some hospitals want a photo ID, such as a driver's license)

- Insurance card

- Insurance or referral forms if required

- List of medicines you take regularly

- Living will and health care power of attorney

- If you will have a hospital stay: clothes and toiletries (toothbrush, toothpaste, and so on)

WHAT HAPPENS DURING THE REGISTRATION AND ADMITTING PROCESS?

This section explains registration and admission for operations other than minor procedures performed in a surgeon's office. Most surgical facilities encourage, or even require, you to preregister a day or more before an elective (scheduled) operation. Advance registration allows you to provide information on your physician, health, and insurance ahead of time. You can preregister on the phone, in person, or sometimes on the hospital's Web site.

The advantage of preregistration is that your wait time will be shorter on the day of your procedure. You may even be able to find out about your financial responsibilities when you preregister if you have not already done so.

In the not-too-distant future, all patients will have an electronic medical record that will include all of this information and that will be transmitted to the hospital before you arrive. So, some day, preregistration may not even be necessary.

Find out where you will need to go on the day of the operation. If you did not preregister, you will probably need to go directly to the surgical facility's admitting office at the scheduled time. An admitting clerk will log your information into the computer system: name, address, referring doctor, surgeon, insurance, and so on.

Some hospitals have found a way to speed registration by issuing patients a computer-readable information card. Such cards have a magnetic strip that contains the patient's name and other pertinent information. A machine electronically reads the data and transmits it to the admitting clerk's computer. After the clerk prints the information, the patient verifies it.

Papers you will need to sign before your operation include a consent form giving your permission to have the operation. Carefully review the consent form before signing it to make sure everything is correct and that you understand it.

You also will need to sign a form saying that you received a HIPAA privacy notice. This document explains how the organization uses your health information and how it keeps identifying information confidential. The federal Health Insurance Portability and Accountability Act of 1996 requires this privacy notice.

For operations using general or intravenous (IV) anesthesia, the admitting clerk or a medical professional will ask when you last ate. If you forgot and ate something, you must tell the people who check you in and your surgeon and anesthesiologist. It may be necessary to reschedule the operation.

After you finish the paperwork, a medical professional (nurse or doctor) will ask you questions about your health. Be prepared to answer questions such as:

• What is your name, and your surgeon's name?

• Do you have any allergies to drugs, foods, or latex?

• What medications do you take? Did you take aspirin recently?

• Do you have a ride home after the procedure?

You may go over these questions more than once with different doctors and hospital staff. Your health care providers check this information for the sake of your safety, so be patient if you must repeat your answers.

If you have any restrictions on treatments (for example, if your religious beliefs do not allow blood transfusions), be sure to mention them.

The medical provider also will perform a brief physical examination. He or she will check your blood pressure, pulse, temperature, heart rate, and breathing.

If you have not already received an identity bracelet, you will be given a wristband with your name on it. It may have other important information, such as your medical record number, birth date, doctor's name, and allergies, if any. Verify that all the information on your ID band is right. Your wristband should be checked by all members of your health care team before doing any procedure or giving you medication.

The admitting process is now done, and you will go to a preoperative area to wait. Hospitals differ on when a family member or friend who came with you can join you and how many people you can have with you in the "preop" area. Ask the staff what the policy is.

WHO WILL TALK TO YOU BEFORE THE OPERATION?

In the preoperative area, nurses or nurse's aides (sometimes called nurse assistants) will be your first point of contact. You will be assigned a bed, and you will change into a hospital gown. If you wear eyeglasses or contact lenses, you will need to remove them before you go to the operating room (OR). A nurse will see that your personal belongings are stored in a safe place. If you are being admitted to the hospital, someone will take your things to your room.

A nurse or other health care provider will start an IV line in a blood vessel in your arm or hand. You will receive fluids and medications through the IV. You also may receive drugs by mouth or by injection. If you are unclear why you are receiving a medication, ask its name and its purpose. For examples of drugs you may receive before anesthesia, see the next section, "What Are These Drugs For?"

Other people you will meet before you go into the OR include your anesthesia provider. This health care professional will review your medical history and answer any questions you have.

Your surgeon may visit you briefly before the procedure. If the surgeon is performing another operation before yours, it may not always be possible to meet with you. If you still have questions for the surgeon, ask to speak with her or him.

What Are These Drugs for?

Medicines that you may get before the operation include:

• A sedative to relax you

• Pain medicine

• An antinausea drug

- Medication to decrease body secretions. Reducing secretions such as saliva and nasal mucus lowers the risk of getting them into your lungs, which may cause pneumonia.

Sometimes antibiotics are given to lessen the chance of an infection at the surgical site. Most operations, however, do not require antibiotics before the procedure. This is a change from the past, when many surgical patients received antibiotics preventively (called antibiotic prophylaxis). Doctors are giving antibiotics less often now, because an overuse of antibiotics is linked to the rise in drug-resistant bacteria.

Today many national medical organizations recommend surgical antibiotic prophylaxis only for procedures that pose an increased risk of bacterial infection. These operations include open heart and certain vascular procedures; colorectal operations; hip and knee joint replacement, spinal disk removal, and other procedures in which a foreign object is implanted; and vaginal or abdominal hysterectomy.

If you do receive an antibiotic shortly before your operation, it may be continued for a short time after the operation.

Of course, you will receive antibiotic treatment if there is already an infection present before an operation, such as in a ruptured appendix.

WILL YOU BE INVOLVED IN MARKING THE SURGICAL SITE?

Everyone has heard news reports about a surgeon operating on the wrong side or area of a patient's body. Fortunately, so-called wrong-site surgical procedures are rare and preventable. To prevent such terrible mistakes from happening, most hospitals and surgical teams now take extra precautions, such as placing an "X" or other mark on the patient's body where the operation should occur. This process is called marking the surgical site.

The American College of Surgeons recognizes patient safety as being of the highest priority. The College has developed suggested guidelines for surgeons and surgical facilities to ensure that the correct procedure is done on the correct site, and on the correct patient.

The College is among many health care organizations that endorsed a safety effort created by The Joint Commission. This project is called the Universal Protocol to Prevent Wrong Site, Wrong Procedure and Wrong Person Surgery. (For more information, visit *www.jointcommission.org/ PatientSafety/SpeakUp.*) The protocol is a requirement for organizations that The Joint Commission accredits.

When to Mark a Surgical Site

The ACS recommends marking the surgical site when an elective procedure involves:

• A bilateral (left- and right-sided) organ, limb (arm or leg), or anatomical site (for example, a breast or hernia)

TAKE CHARGE OF YOUR SAFETY

Patients should take an active role in helping ensure that they have an error-free operation. Here are some tips:

• Allow only the spot being operated on to be marked. Writing "no" on the other side can be confusing.

• Site marking should occur before you receive narcotic painkillers, sedation, or anesthesia. If that is not possible, ask a family member or friend to make sure the surgeon correctly marks the site.

• Carefully read the consent form before you sign it. Make sure it correctly states what the operation is and where on the body it is to be performed.

• Make sure the surgical team member asks your name or checks your ID bracelet before marking the site.

• Ask the surgeon if she or he will remain with you from beginning to end of the operation.

- Multiple structures (such as fingers or toes)

- Multiple levels (as in the spine)

The surgeon or another member of the surgical team should mark the patient's skin at the surgical site with an indelible marker or pen (one that won't wash off right away). If not, ask for the correct location to be marked.

Some surgical facilities may ask the patient to mark the site. But The Joint Commission does not recommend this approach, because many patients do not mark the site as instructed. You should, however, be involved by agreeing on the site that the surgeon will mark.

Marking the surgical site is not required if there is an obvious wound being repaired or if the operation is an emergency.

INSIDER'S TIP

A time-out is a final safety check in the OR before the operation begins. Once you are on the operating table, a surgical team member states the name of the patient, the type of procedure to be performed, and the surgical site. The operation should not start until the surgeon and other team members agree that this information is correct. They will make sure that the name on your ID bracelet matches the one on the consent form and any medical images, such as X rays, are available in the OR.

Similar to the safety inspection pilots do before flying, a surgical time-out also allows the OR team to ensure they have all the needed equipment in place. During the pause, the surgical team also discusses the patient's special needs, if there are any.

This verification process may happen before or after you receive anesthesia. Ask your surgeon if there will be a time-out to discuss your case and whether he or she will participate in the time-out. I made sure to ask my surgeon about this procedure before my gallbladder operation!

WILL SOMEONE GO OVER WHAT WILL BE DONE DURING THE OPERATION?

Before you sign a consent form, someone from the surgical team should review with you what will happen during the procedure.

Every operation is different, so I can't give specifics on your particular procedure. But there are some things that are common to most operations.

Most of the time, you will be sedated before you go into the OR. You will be brought into the OR on a bed with wheels or in a wheelchair. Before you go into the OR, you may wait briefly in a holding area while the OR team makes the room ready for your operation. It may be in this holding area that you see your surgeon for the first time that day.

Getting "Prepped" for a Surgical Procedure

Once you are in the OR and under anesthesia, the surgical team will prepare ("prep" in surgical slang) you for the operation.

Your anesthesia professional will not allow an operation to start before all the monitors are on and working (measuring your heart rate, blood pressure, breathing rate, temperature, and so on). Your anesthesia provider will stay with you in the OR throughout your procedure.

If you receive general anesthesia, you probably will receive a breathing tube. (Sometimes the patient wears an anesthesia mask instead.) This insertion of a tube into the trachea, or windpipe, is called intubation. A breathing tube is needed because many anesthetic medications slow down or stop patients' ability to breathe on their own. (You'll be relieved to hear that as soon as you begin to wake up, the breathing tube is removed.)

You may be given other tubes or a catheter—a tube—to remove body fluids such as urine. You will receive intravenous fluids during the operation through your IV. Fluids prevent dehydration and help your liver and kidneys to metabolize (process) the anesthetic medicine.

Infection Control Starts Before the Operation

Operations take place behind closed doors to keep the OR as sterile as possible. Before the surgeon makes an incision, an antibacterial medicated solution will be applied to the surgical site to clean it. Then the OR team will drape sterile coverings over your body except for the surgical site.

Most modern ORs use these preparations as well as special air-flow systems, and all members of the surgical team wear sterile gowns over their scrub clothes, gloves, and masks. All of these things—plus thorough hand washing by the surgical team—are done to minimize the chance of contamination.

When the surgical wound or an organ or body space entered during the operation becomes infected, it is called a surgical-site infection. These infections are a major source of postoperative illness and can even be life-threatening. Therefore, surgical teams take many steps to try to prevent infection. In addition to the sterile OR procedures just mentioned, these efforts include:

- The appropriate use of antibiotics

- Cutting or clipping hair in the surgical area, rather than shaving it, which can cause nicks in the skin and lead to infection

- Ensuring that skin and tissues get adequate oxygen during and after the operation, which improves wound healing

- Controlling body temperature and glucose levels (see "Insider's Tip," page 58)

Preventing Blood Clots

When you have an operation, your need to remain in bed for an extended period of time puts you at risk for developing blood clots in your legs. The longer and more complicated your operation, the greater this risk. Your surgeon will know your risks and take steps to prevent them. Preventive measures may include blood-thinning medication and support or compression stockings.

HOW LONG WILL THE OPERATION LAST?

Of course, you will want to know how long you will be in the OR. Bear in mind, however, that your surgeon will give you only an estimate of

INSIDER'S TIP

Abnormally low body temperature in the OR may increase your risk of an infection developing at the surgical site. Warming a patient before the operation can prevent body temperature from going too low in the OR. Surgical facilities use warming systems or heated blankets to keep patients warm. So if you are cold in the preoperative area, tell a nurse.

Make sure the surgical team will keep you warm during the operation if it will last more than an hour. Ask if they will monitor your temperature.

If you are diabetic, make sure that the OR staff will monitor your blood glucose (sugar) level. If it becomes too high, a surgical-site infection could develop. Blood glucose control is important!

the length of the procedure. There are many reasons why an operation may last longer than your surgeon estimated. It does not necessarily mean that there were complications. For example, if you are overweight or you have had past operations in this area and have scar tissue there, it is more time-consuming for the surgeon to perform the operation.

Often, if an operation is taking much longer than estimated, the hospital staff will inform your family.

WILL THE SURGEON TALK TO YOUR FAMILY AFTER THE OPERATION?

After the procedure is over, your surgeon will briefly talk to your family member or other individual you have designated as a contact. The surgeon will tell them how the operation went and answer any questions.

Here are some questions your family or friend may want to ask the surgeon:

• Was the operation successful?

- Why did the operation take longer than you thought it would?

- Did anything unexpected happen during the operation?

- Did the patient lose a lot of blood?

- How long will the patient be in the recovery room? In the hospital?

- Is there anything that could complicate the patient's recovery?

- Has there been any change in the postoperative plans?

HOW LONG WILL YOU BE IN RECOVERY?

After the operation, most patients who have had anesthesia are transferred to a recovery room. It sometimes is called the postanesthesia care unit, or PACU. This area is where you recover from the immediate effects of anesthesia. Some patients who are admitted to the hospital go directly to their rooms or, if they need close monitoring, to the Intensive Care Unit (ICU).

How long you stay in recovery depends on the type of anesthesia you were given and whether you have a history of medical problems. Most patients stay about an hour.

As the anesthetic wears off, your anesthesia provider oversees your safe recovery. Specially trained nurses in the recovery room will closely monitor your heart rate, breathing rate, blood pressure, and oxygen saturation.

Oxygen saturation is the percentage of hemoglobin saturation in your blood. Hemoglobin is the protein in red blood cells that transports oxygen to tissues. The oxygen saturation shows how well your lungs are providing oxygen to the blood. The device that measures oxygen saturation is typically a pulse oximeter. It is inserted over a fingertip (or less often an earlobe or toe). It looks somewhat like a clothespin, but it doesn't hurt. Patients often receive extra oxygen in recovery.

In some surgical facilities, you will be brought to another area, where you will continue to recover. The person or persons who took you to the hospital may be allowed to join you at this point, and you will begin to wake up if you did not do so in the recovery room.

WHAT IS FAST-TRACK SURGERY, AND WILL YOU HAVE IT?

Many operations today are done on a fast track. Operations are quicker. Patients stay in the hospital a shorter time, or the procedure is done on an outpatient basis. Patients receive shorter-acting anesthetics, and they are asked to get up from bed sooner. Hospitals use care plans designed to optimize outcomes, reduce the risk of complications, and shorten the length of stay. Pain control sometimes starts before the operation, so that patients may have minimal pain.

In short, recovery is faster.

The use of minimally invasive operations has helped reduce postoperative recovery time. Recovery also is quicker thanks to advances in pain control, anesthesia, and postoperative care. In addition, medical professionals better understand how to reduce the body's stress response due to the surgical procedure.

When an operation involves a combination of techniques to reduce the surgical stress response and to shorten recovery time, it is called fast-track surgery. It may go by other names, such as rapid recovery. Whatever the name, most surgeons are using fast-track techniques to some extent.

A fast-track approach uses the same discharge criteria as those of traditional care but achieves the criteria sooner.

A PATIENT'S PERSPECTIVE

Nancy Weissenstein, 62-year-old who had cataract operations in 2006

"If you don't want surprises, ask a lot of questions. I'm a surgical technician—a scrub nurse—but it's different being the patient. I had lots of questions for the surgeon about my first cataract surgery. You should not be any less informed because you're having outpatient surgery."

Fast-tracking is based on evidence from studies in patients. For many procedures, studies comparing the fast-track approach with conventional treatment have shown these benefits of the fast track:

- Shorter hospital stay

- Less pain and fatigue

- Faster ability to walk and resume normal activities

- Improved or similar patient satisfaction

Researchers continue to study the benefits of fast-track surgery and whether there are any increased risks to the patient.

Patient education is an important part of the success of fast-track surgery. Ask your surgeon if your operation will be done on a fast track, and what that means for you. Feel free to discuss any concerns you have with your surgeon.

What to Ask the Surgeon

☐ What should I bring to the surgical facility?

☐ What happens during the registration and admitting process?

☐ Who will talk to me before the operation?

☐ Will I be involved in marking the surgical site?

☐ Will someone go over what will be done during the operation?

☐ How long will the operation last?

☐ Will the surgeon talk to my family after the operation?

☐ How long will I be in recovery?

☐ What is fast-track surgery, and will I have it?

SIX

After the Operation

IN THIS CHAPTER

- Pain relief: What every surgical patient wants to know

- What happens if you need a hospital stay or intensive care

- Why you have to get moving before you feel ready

- How to avoid being the victim of a medication error

- What to ask the surgeon

HOW WILL YOU FEEL AFTER THE OPERATION?

As you can see from the preceding comments from actual patients, postoperative experiences can run the gamut. How patients feel in the hours and weeks after an operation can range from having little or no discomfort to having severe pain, fatigue, and other problems—or somewhere in between.

My own recent experience with having an outpatient gallbladder operation is that the postoperative recovery is the hardest part of an operation. By the third day after the operation, the anesthesia and pain medications I received in the hospital had worn off, and the surgical site (on my abdomen) hurt. My sleep cycle was disrupted, and I slept a lot for the first week.

What I found, and what many other surgical patients discover, is that usually you feel worse before you feel better.

For an operation to succeed, you must heal. Yet during the first few

A PATIENT'S PERSPECTIVE

Margaret Telow, 46-year-old who had both hips replaced in 2005

"My recovery was hard. I did six hours of physical therapy every day while I was in the hospital. After I went home, I had severe swelling in my lower legs. I was out of work four months."

Nancy Weissenstein, 62-year-old who had cataracts removed from both eyes in 2006

"My cataract operations were a very easy experience for me. I had no problems afterward, and there was no pain or discomfort. I went back to work within two days. I had my right eye operated on first and then two weeks later, the left eye. By four weeks, I had 20/20 vision."

Dave Davis, 70-year-old who in 1996 had a carotid endarterectomy, a vascular surgical procedure to remove plaque blocking a carotid artery in his neck, and thus prevent a stroke

"It took a while to recover from the operation and get my energy back. I felt weak, and I slept a lot. My surgeon said that was normal and not to push it. It was hard for me, because I wanted to get going right away. I'm a type A personality. But my body told me otherwise. It was two weeks before I felt like coming back to the office, and I went back part time at first."

days after the operation, very little healing occurs. Be patient. An operation is a major stress on your body, and healing is physically and emotionally draining. Healing can take three to six months or longer to be complete.

Why Recovery Time Varies

Your recovery and how you'll feel after your operation will depend on many factors. They include:

- Type of operation and area of body operated on

- Surgical approach (faster recovery for minimally invasive procedures)

- Type of anesthesia

- Your pain tolerance

- Your general health

- Your anxiety level (anxiety contributes to postoperative pain)

- How well you follow your health care team's instructions or treatment plan and your active involvement in carrying out that plan

Treatment Plan

Some hospitals give patients a written day-to-day treatment plan. Treatment plans generally identify the health care team's goals for treatment and the methods for achieving the goals. A treatment plan also includes expectations of what the patient needs to do to get well. It is a huge motivator for the patient to know the health care team's expectations.

Even if you do not receive a treatment plan in writing, your care team will give you postoperative instructions. It is important to follow these instructions because they are designed to get you well faster.

Private or Semiprivate Room

If you need a hospital stay and believe you will recover better with quiet and privacy, ask ahead of time for a private room (one bed). Most new hospitals have private rooms, and some older hospitals are converting their inpatient floors to all private rooms. Many, however, still have semi-private rooms (two beds). There may be an extra cost for a private room that your insurance plan will not cover.

Aftereffects

This chapter deals primarily with recovery immediately after an operation, while you are in the hospital or surgical center. The last chapter discusses recovery after you go home.

So, how will you feel right after the operation?

When you first wake up after the operation is over, you may have a dry mouth from the medicine that stopped your saliva and mucus production. You also may have a sore or scratchy throat if you had a breathing tube in your throat during the operation. (It is removed before you wake up.)

You may feel nauseated or may vomit because of the anesthesia you received. However, vomiting is becoming less frequent with advances in anesthetics and antinausea drugs. Most patients feel groggy when the anesthesia starts to wear off. Some people feel disoriented or have blurred vision. Having chills is also possible. These are temporary effects of the anesthetic drugs.

Patients usually feel some discomfort and pain at the surgical site. Thus, pain control is an important part of recovery in the hours and days after an operation.

WHAT ABOUT PAIN RELIEF?

One of the most common fears about having an operation is feeling pain. Fortunately, health care providers do their best to minimize pain and make patients comfortable after an operation. Some hospitals even have a team of doctors and nurses who are specially trained in analgesia, as health care providers call pain management.

Doctors better understand pain today. Studies have shown that proper pain management helps patients recover more quickly and with fewer complications. *The bottom line is, pain can be controlled today. No patient should ever be in severe pain.*

Sometimes pain control starts before or during the surgical procedure! Before postoperative pain even begins, doctors may give some patients an injection of a long-lasting pain medicine. This type of pre-emptive pain control is new. Its effectiveness in reducing postsurgical pain varies with the type of procedure, however. Sometimes it improves pain relief, and sometimes it does not.

It is more typical for pain control to begin after a procedure, but even this approach has changed. Health care providers no longer wait to give pain relief until pain is bad. That's because severe pain is harder to control. After your operation, don't wait for your pain to get bad. Tell your doctor or nurse as soon as you start to have pain.

To determine your level of pain, doctors and nurses will ask you to rate your pain on a scale of 0 to 10. A score of 0 indicates no pain, and 10 is the worst possible pain.

Types of Pain Control

The painkillers most often used immediately after an operation are narcotics, such as fentanyl, morphine, codeine, and oxycodone. Narcotics (also called opioids) control severe or moderate pain.

Narcotics may be combined with acetaminophen (Tylenol) or a nonsteroidal anti-inflammatory drug (NSAID), such as aspirin, ibuprofen, or naproxen. If your pain is mild or you are allergic to narcotics, you may receive just NSAIDs. You will not receive NSAIDs, however, if you are at risk of postoperative bleeding.

Pain medicine may be given through an intravenous (IV) catheter, injected into a muscle or skin, given orally in pill or liquid form, or dripped into the surgical wound (called a local anesthetic). Sometimes the surgeon injects a local anesthetic, such as lidocaine, into the surgical wound at the time of the operation. In some cases, pain medication may also be given through an epidural, an injection in the spine.

Not all pain control involves medication. Patients also may wish to listen to relaxation tapes or use other relaxation techniques to cope with pain and anxiety.

If your incision is on your stomach or chest, it will help reduce pain when you cough if you hold a pillow against the area.

Drug Side Effects

Side effects of narcotics include:

- severe drowsiness

- constipation

- stomach upset or vomiting

- skin rash or itching

- lowered blood pressure, which can cause dizziness, especially when getting up

Sometimes people are allergic to some narcotic medicines. Medications are available to control many of the side effects of narcotics, so let your surgeon know if you experience any. It is often recommended that you increase the fiber in your diet, which helps produce regular bowel movements if you are constipated.

Don't let concerns about addiction to strong pain medications like narcotics keep you from taking the drugs the surgeon prescribed to help you heal comfortably. Research shows that becoming addicted to pain medication after an operation is extremely rare.

Side effects of short-term use of NSAIDs include stomach pain, heartburn, increased postoperative bleeding, and allergic reactions, such as a rash. These side effects are usually not seen with short-term use. NSAIDs are not addictive.

In the Hospital

If you are staying in the hospital, the IV catheter inserted in your arm or hand before the operation probably will be left in place. That way, you can get your pain medicine and IV fluids through it.

In the hospital, you may have a patient-controlled analgesia (PCA) pump. When you push a button on this computerized pump, it injects pain medicine into your IV. Because the amount is limited to the prescribed dose, you cannot give yourself too much pain medicine.

Another way to receive IV pain medicine in the hospital is for a nurse to put the drug directly into your IV catheter. If you have a PCA pump, it will be stopped when your pain lessens and you are nearly ready to go home, and the IV may be removed. Then you will receive oral pain medicine. Often this medicine is a narcotic. The goal is to get you on oral pain medicine as soon as possible. Let your nurse know as soon as you start to feel pain because the oral medication takes a little longer to work than the IV medication does.

WILL YOU BE IN INTENSIVE CARE?

For a procedure involving a hospital stay, ask if you will need to spend time in the intensive care unit (ICU). Sometimes called the critical care unit, the ICU is a special unit where patients receive close monitoring and extra care. Some patients may need to go to the ICU immediately after a major operation, although most patients don't require intensive care. Most often you'll know ahead of time if you'll need an ICU stay.

A stay in the ICU is typical after complex operations, such as open heart and brain surgical procedures. Open heart surgical patients generally stay in the coronary care unit, where they receive intensive care.

You also may spend time in the ICU if you need a ventilator (also called respirator)—a machine to help you breathe.

Equipment commonly used in the ICU includes:

- Cardiac and respiratory monitor—You will have wires attached to your chest that will monitor the electrical activity of your heart and your breathing pattern.

- Oxygen saturation monitor—A sensor that will be placed on your finger to monitor the oxygen in your blood.

- Oxygen—Oxygen may be given through a mask on your face, through nasal prongs, or by a ventilator.

- Other equipment in an ICU may include an arterial line. This device is a thin catheter inserted into an artery—a type of blood vessel—most often in the wrist or groin. The purpose of this line is to constantly monitor blood pressure. Blood samples also can be taken from an arterial line to monitor oxygen saturation—how well the lungs are providing oxygen to the blood.

In the ICU, you will have a nurse who is trained in intensive care. There is typically one nurse for every one to three patients, depending on how severe the patient's condition is. Ask your surgeon before a hospital stay what the ICU's nurse-to-patient ratio is. You want to make sure you will receive proper attention.

In some hospital ICUs, you may receive care from an intensivist, a physician trained in critical care medicine and surgery. This doctor can be a surgeon, an anesthesiologist, a pulmonologist (lung specialist), or other physician.

When your condition becomes more stable, you will be moved from the ICU to a regular medical-surgical nursing floor in the hospital, before going home.

WILL YOU BE HOOKED UP TO ANY MACHINES IN THE HOSPITAL?

If you do not spend time in an ICU, you probably will be hooked up to only one machine: an IV pump, also called an infusion pump. This pump hangs on a stand with wheels. It runs on batteries when it is unplugged. Your IV may be used to give IV medications and fluids.

Patients who are on bed rest will need to wear compression or support stockings. Compression stockings are connected to an air compressor. The compressor inflates and deflates compartments in plastic wraps around the stockings. The gentle pressure on the leg muscles when you're lying down, and unable to move, decreases the chance of a blood clot forming. You should leave these stockings on as long as your care providers tell you to. Your surgeon may choose to put you on a blood-thinning medication, which is also used to decrease your risk of developing clots.

Breathe Deeply

Developing pneumonia is a risk after an operation because of general anesthesia and lack of movement. To prevent lung infection, your health care team will ask you to breathe deeply and cough every few hours.

Movement and deep breathing after your operation can help prevent fluid from collecting in your lungs, which can lead to the development of pneumonia. An effective way to do deep breathing is to take a deep breath and hold it for three to five seconds. Take two to 10 deep breaths every hour while you are awake. Young children can do deep breathing by blowing bubbles or balloons.

As a stimulus to breathe more deeply, you may be given a handheld device called an incentive spirometer. It has numbers on it that show how much air you are moving through your lungs. To use it, breathe out and place your lips firmly around the mouthpiece. Breathe in slowly and deeply. Hold your breath for about five seconds. Then remove your lips and exhale. Your nurse will tell you how often to repeat these steps.

Abdominal Operations

One other postoperative problem is worth mentioning here. Any abdominal operation can cause a temporary paralysis of the bowels (also called intestines). Doctors call this inability to move the bowels paralytic ileus. (It occurs less often with laparoscopy than with open procedures.) Symptoms are stomach pain and bloating, constipation, loss of appetite or nausea, and vomiting. This problem usually lasts two or three days.

The patient is not allowed to eat or drink anything until bowel function returns. Other treatment may be needed if the patient is very uncomfortable or the ileus continues. On occasion, the person will need a suction tube placed down the nose to the stomach. This nasogastric tube suctions fluid from the stomach and gets the bowels working again.

Less often after an abdominal operation, the bowels become physically blocked. A mechanical blockage of the intestines can occur soon after an abdominal operation or, more commonly, at any time in the future. It results later from scar tissue (called adhesions) forming inside the abdomen. The bowels can even become twisted from adhesions, and another operation may be needed.

Symptoms of a postoperative intestinal obstruction are similar to those of paralytic ileus. Doctors diagnose bowel obstruction and paralytic ileus through a physical exam and sometimes X ray of the abdomen or another imaging test.

WHEN WILL YOUR SURGEON VISIT YOU?

Your surgeon will first visit you in the recovery room, but you probably won't remember it! If you are staying in the hospital, your surgeon or an associate will visit you that first night and every day after that until your discharge.

WHO ELSE WILL BE TAKING CARE OF YOU?

Many other health care providers will take care of you in the hospital. Depending on your condition, you may need care from physician specialists. Other physicians who may treat you include hospitalists. These doctors specialize in treating hospitalized patients.

If you are in a teaching hospital, you will receive care from doctors in training, under the supervision of an experienced attending physician. Medical doctors who are training in a specialty of medicine, such as general surgery, are called residents. Physicians who are getting more advanced training after their residency are known as fellows.

The health care professionals you most often will meet are nurses and nurse assistants (also called aides). Nurses give you the medicines and other treatments your doctor orders, examine you, and record your progress. Nurses may be registered nurses (RNs), licensed practical nurses (LPNs), or licensed vocational nurses (LVNs). LPNs and LVNs perform basic levels of care at the patient's bedside and report to an RN. An RN is trained to both give and plan patient care. The RN who is in charge of nursing care on the hospital floor is called the charge nurse.

Like doctors, nurses may have more advanced training. A nurse practitioner is an advanced-practice nurse with a master's degree. Typically, a nurse practitioner has more responsibilities than a nurse. In some states, a nurse practitioner can prescribe medicine.

A clinical nurse specialist is a nurse with a master's degree who specializes in one area of nursing (for example, cancer treatment).

Nurse assistants (also called patient care assistants or nurse's aides) help nurses. They change your sheets, help you bathe, and take your blood pressure and temperature.

Other health care workers in the hospital include:

- Rehabilitation therapists, such as physical, occupational, respiratory, or speech therapists

- Phlebotomist (someone trained to draw blood)

- Technicians, who perform tests

- Physician's assistant (a care provider, usually not a nurse, who is trained to help a doctor and works under the doctor's supervision)

- Dietitian

- Social worker

- Chaplain

- Discharge planner (may be a nurse, social worker, or other professional)

Now that you have a better idea of how many people are on a health care team, you can probably see why being in a hospital is so expensive!

WHAT CAN YOU DO TO PREVENT MEDICATION ERRORS?

Medication errors can occur in hospitals and surgical facilities, sometimes with grave consequences. However, hospitals and health care providers are working to improve medication safety. Some hospitals have adopted new ways of protecting patients from receiving the wrong drug or wrong dose. Examples include:

- "Smart" drug infusion pumps that have computer software with built-in safety checks that warn of medication errors

- Computer alerts that send a notice from the hospital's lab to its pharmacy if a patient's medication levels are outside appropriate limits on lab results

- Medication reconciliation programs to make sure that all hospital departments correctly communicate a patient's medication information when the patient is admitted, transferred to another unit, or discharged.

- Bar codes on medications that must be matched to a bar code on the patient's ID bracelet

    You, too, can do things to help avoid mistakes happening with your medications or with doses being missed.

- When a nurse or doctor brings you a new medicine, ask what it is for, who prescribed it, how often you'll get it, and what its side effects are.

- Read the name on any bag of IV fluid or medication you receive, or ask someone else to read it.

- Make sure that the care provider checks your ID bracelet or asks your name before giving you medication.

- If you don't receive your medicine when you think you are supposed to, tell a nurse.

- Don't be afraid to tell a nurse or doctor if you think you are about to be given the wrong drug.

- Tell your nurse right away if you have a bad reaction or don't feel well after receiving medicine.

- If you bring your own medicines to the hospital give them to the nurse. Do not take them without the nurse's supervision because doing so may interfere with another drug you are receiving. Instead, ask your surgeon to prescribe it for you. Note: Many hospitals encourage patients to bring their meds. As hospital pharmacies get more and more restrictive, a patient may be asked to take a different but equally effective drug. Ask your surgeon. He or she may give an order for you to take your own medicine to avoid making a change.

- Remember your patient rights (see pages 9-10). You have the right to review your medical record. If you have any questions or concerns about your medications or other treatment, ask to see your patient chart.

INSIDER'S TIP

Here's another safety tip. To prevent infection, make sure that all care providers wash their hands before, or wear gloves while, they check, wash, or bandage your surgical wound. Feel free to ask them to wash their hands if you don't see them do so, or to wear gloves. Protection against infection is especially important if your immune system is compromised—for example, if you have received chemotherapy.

WHEN CAN YOU GET OUT OF BED?

It's not a matter of when you can, but rather when you should, get out of bed. The answer to that is as soon as possible.

Patients used to be told to lie in bed for a week after a surgical procedure. For most operations today, you'll be asked to get up, bear weight, and start moving the part of your body that was operated on by the morning of the first postoperative day. Sometimes the nurses in the hospital will encourage you to get up on the night of the day you have the operation, even if it's just sitting up and putting your legs over the side of the bed.

Why the change to early movement and walking ("ambulation")? Simply put, it speeds your recovery. There are multiple benefits to all organs in your body. It improves function and gets your body back into a normal routine quickly. Early movement also gets your digestive tract moving. Finally, it prevents blood clots from forming

You need to get up and move around a little, even though it hurts. (You'll receive pain medicine shortly before your nurse gets you up.) Slowly build your activity level every day.

In some cases, your surgeon may want to limit your movement right after the operation. That may be the case because you are weak or receiving medicine that causes dizziness, or after procedures that affect mobility, such as joint replacement.

Bladder Catheter

Sometimes patients receive a urinary bladder catheter while they are in the operating room. You may receive a catheter in any of these situations:

- You have, or are expected to have, difficulty getting up to go to the bathroom.

- You had a bladder, pelvis, or prostate operation, which may make it hard to urinate, and you are given a catheter for the first day or two.

- Your doctor needs to measure your urine output hourly, to decide how much IV fluid to give you after an extensive operation. (Even if you don't have a catheter, your urine output may still need to be measured. You would then be asked to urinate in a cup or other container.)

Urine will drip from the catheter into a drainage bag. Someone on your health care team will empty the bag when it becomes full.

It is important to know that you will not be able to feel the catheter once it is in place.

WHEN CAN YOU RESUME A NORMAL DIET?

Just like walking, patients are beginning to eat sooner after an operation. It's all part of fast-track surgery, to shorten recovery time (see Chapter 5 on page 60). Eating early after an operation appears to be safe and, some studies show, also beneficial. As always, however, ask your surgeon.

When you eat and what you eat will depend on the type of operation and your response to anesthesia. To lessen the chance of throwing up after anesthesia, you will first receive ice chips and small amounts of clear liquids to drink. When you can tolerate that, you will be given soft foods and then a regular diet. Some patients will be able to eat solid foods without trying soft foods first.

In my practice of colon surgery, I asked my patients what they wanted to eat if they were doing well. They were in the best position to know when they could eat. But be sure to check with your surgeon.

Eat when you feel ready to eat. And eat what you can; don't feel obligated to eat all the food on the tray.

Bear in mind that low-fat foods are easier to digest than fried and other high-fat foods. For digestive, weight-loss, or colon operations, your surgeon may recommend foods you should avoid eating and set limits on the amount you can eat.

If you have food allergies or restrictions, be sure to tell your nurse. Also, write them on your menu order for the food service staff.

INSIDER'S TIP

My advice, if you need a hospital stay, is to have realistic expectations about the loss of privacy and personal control in the hospital. Some hospitalized patients feel like they've been stripped of a part of themselves by this lack of control.

In the hospital, you have constant reminders that you are not at home. You're told when to eat, you may not have much of a choice in what to eat, and it's not fine dining, to be sure! You are awakened several times during the night to have your vital signs measured, so you can't sleep when you want to. Hospitals try to control noise levels, but a hospital is still a noisy place. You're treated by a lot of people you don't know. You wear a hospital gown with your back exposed, and you may lose your modesty quickly.

It helps to accept that there are some things about the surgical experience that you cannot control. But you can regain some of your personal control by actively participating in your recovery. Try to eat properly, move around as instructed, and do your deep breathing and coughing. After all, you want this operation to succeed, so you won't have to go through it again!

WHEN CAN YOU GO HOME?

Before you can safely go home ("be discharged"), you will need to meet certain criteria.

Discharge Criteria

The discharge criteria for a surgical procedure may include, among others:

- Being awake

- Stable vital signs

- Ability to drink fluids and maintain adequate hydration (usually about two liters of water or its equivalent per day)

- Ability to resume walking with help

- Ability to urinate or have a catheter in place

- Pain adequately controlled

- Ability to function at home (eat, get up, and so on) or have assistance with daily activities

Before discharge, the surgeon or a doctor your surgeon designates will examine you to make sure you are ready to leave. Only a doctor can order a discharge.

Your surgeon may transfer you to another health care facility instead of sending you home. You may need to go to another facility if you need continued nursing care or rehabilitation, or more help than someone at home can provide. If you need to go to an extended-care facility, make sure it is accredited.

Discharge Instructions

The nurses and your surgeon will teach you and your family home care and give you any special instructions in writing before you leave the hospital. Examples include:

- Names and a schedule of doses of medications you will take, and their side effects

- What you can eat and what you should avoid

- How to take care of the surgical wound, how often to change the bandage, and how to look for signs of infection

- When you can shower or bathe

- What activities you shouldn't do, and when you can resume doing them

- If needed, how to use special equipment (crutches, walker, catheter, feeding tube, oxygen machine, etc.)

- When you should schedule a follow-up visit with your surgeon

- Whether you need home health care

- What symptoms you should watch for and when and how to contact your surgeon. Usually you will be instructed to call your surgeon for:
  - Pain that will not go away
  - Pain that gets worse
  - A fever that is more than 101°F
  - Continuous vomiting
  - Swelling, redness, bleeding, or bad smelling drainage from an incision site

Make sure you understand all the instructions before you go home.

If the hospital wants to discharge you and you do not feel well enough to go home, ask to speak to your surgeon. Only your surgeon can order your discharge. He or she may request that you go to an extended-care facility or receive home care.

Don't worry if you're leaving the hospital and you have not yet had a bowel movement. Inpatients must no longer wait until their bowel function returns to be discharged. Doctors know that the return of this function can take some time and that patients will feel more comfortable going to the bathroom at home.

When you are discharged—whether as an inpatient or outpatient—you will not be allowed to drive yourself home. Plan on getting a ride.

WHAT SHOULD YOU DO IF YOU HAVE CONCERNS?

If you have any concerns about your recovery or treatment, speak to your surgeon. Make sure, before you go home, that you have your surgeon's contact information.

During a hospital stay, you also can speak to your nurse about concerns related to your care.

For help with financial arrangements or referral to community resources, the hospital social worker is the best person to contact.

If you have a conflict with a care provider, ask to speak with another care provider or a hospital representative. Many hospitals have a patient representative or patient liaison, who is there to act on your behalf. He or she will act as a go-between with the care provider and will try to smooth out the difficulties.

What to Ask the Surgeon

☐ How will I feel after the operation?

☐ What will the affected part of my body look like?

☐ What kinds of devices or machines will I be hooked up to?

☐ What about pain relief?

☐ When can I get out of bed?

☐ When can I resume a normal diet?

☐ When can I go home?

☐ What should I do if I have concerns?

If I need a hospital stay:

☐ Will I be in intensive care?

☐ Will I be hooked up to any machines in the hospital?

☐ When will you visit me?

☐ Who else will be taking care of me?

☐ What can I do to prevent medication errors?

SEVEN

After You Go Home

IN THIS CHAPTER

- Possible complications, and what to do if they happen

- Resuming normal activities

- Getting stitches removed

- Home care and other treatment

- What to ask the surgeon

Most of your recovery will occur at home.

WHAT ABOUT PAIN RELIEF?

When you leave the hospital, you'll rely on oral medications for pain control. (For inpatients who are receiving medicine intravenously, the hospital staff will change your pain medicine to pills or another oral form before you go home.)

Make sure you know the name of the medication (generic and brand name) and how often to take it. If you have had pain medicine in the past that worked for you, ask your surgeon for that drug.

Find out if the pain medicine your surgeon prescribes contains acetaminophen (also known as the brand name Tylenol®). If it does, do not take acetaminophen at the same time as your prescription pain medicine. Be careful that you do not take more than the recommended dose of acetaminophen, which can harm the liver.

The surgeon may prescribe narcotic (opioid) painkillers after the operation. Your pain should get a little better soon after your operation, so take your pain medicine less often when your pain begins to lessen. If your pain gets worse, there is probably something wrong. Call your surgeon.

If you use narcotics for a long time, your body will develop a tolerance for the medicine, meaning you will need more of it to get the same effect. This is a normal situation for narcotics, so don't worry about it. As you start feeling better, you will start to decrease the dose.

Nonnarcotic options are acetaminophen or nonsteroidal anti-inflammatory drugs (NSAIDs), such as ibuprofen, naproxen, and aspirin.

Alcohol and Painkillers Don't Mix

One side effect of narcotics is they cause drowsiness and fatigue. Do not drive or operate machines while you are taking a narcotic. Also avoid alcohol because it will increase the drowsy effect. Don't take sedating drugs such as antihistamines or sedatives in addition to a narcotic unless your doctor recommends them.

Do not drink alcohol while taking acetaminophen. Taken together, they can damage the liver.

Prevent Constipation

Narcotics can also be constipating. It's a good idea to take a stool softener while you are taking narcotic painkillers. Here are other ways you can prevent constipation:

- Drink prune juice, a natural laxative.

- Drink plenty of water.

- Try to get enough fiber in your diet, or use an over-the-counter fiber supplement. Foods that contain a lot of fiber include whole-grain breads and cereals, fruits and vegetables, and beans and peas.

- Limit the fried and high-fat foods you eat, as they can cause constipation.

- Get up and move around every day. Not getting enough exercise can cause constipation.

WHAT SHOULD YOU DO ABOUT BLEEDING OR OTHER PROBLEMS?

No surgical procedure is free of risks. There are no guarantees that there won't be any complications. Despite every effort to prevent problems, sometimes complications occur. Fortunately, they are fairly rare.

As discussed throughout this book, you can help minimize the chance of developing complications by actions you take before and after the operation. Follow your surgeon's instructions, eat properly, get enough exercise, and stop smoking.

Call Your Surgeon

Possible complications after any operation, and their symptoms, are listed in the table on page 84. If you experience any of the problems listed in the table or you have worsening pain, call your surgeon's office. Explain your symptoms to a nurse and ask to speak with the doctor as soon as possible.

Go to the emergency room if you have chest pain or difficulty breathing.

These problems are less urgent but if they persist, let your surgeon know:

- Constipation (inability to move your bowels)

- Fluid retention (as shown by ankle swelling or steep weight gain)

- Lack of appetite (inability to eat due to nausea and vomiting)

- Dehydration (dark-colored or strong smelling urine or a decrease in volume of your urine)

- Need for more pain medicine or a change in pain medicine

- Depression lasting longer than two weeks

- Persistent fever, especially if accompanied by chills

Most of the time, you need not be concerned about a low-grade fever (temperature of 99°F to 100.9°F). A slightly high body temperature is common after an operation and generally is not serious. A fever is the body's natural response to fighting an infection or illness. Drink plenty of fluids so you won't become dehydrated. Ask your doctor before taking fever-reducing medication, such as acetaminophen (Tylenol®) or aspirin.

MOST COMMON POSTOPERATIVE COMPLICATIONS	
COMPLICATION	SYMPTOMS AND SIGNS*
Severe bleeding (occurs most often in the first few days after an operation)	**External:** Severe bleeding from the wound **Internal:** Indicated by pain; pale, clammy skin; increased heart rate; weakness; mental confusion; black-and-blue bruises; blood in the stool or urine
Wound infection	Redness, swelling, or heat around the surgical wound; pus from the wound; high fever (103°F and above)
Blood clots in a leg	Pain, swelling, or redness in one leg
Pneumonia	Chest pain that worsens with coughing or deep breathing; shortness of breath; cough with green or yellow discharge; fever with chills
Bladder infection (if you had a urinary catheter)	Pain or burning when you urinate; frequent need to urinate; cloudy or bloody urine or urine that smells bad; pressure in the lower abdomen; fever

*Tell your doctor about these.

Each surgical procedure also has its own potential complications besides those listed in the table. Your health care team will give you written information about warning signs of complications before you leave the surgical facility.

A Warning for Smokers

If you smoke, try to quit. Smoking is detrimental to healing and can lead to complications.

WHEN CAN YOU RESUME NORMAL ACTIVITIES?

For a certain time after a major operation while you heal, you likely will have some restriction in activities. Activities you may not be able to do for a certain time include driving, working, lifting or pushing anything heavy, bending, exercising, and bathing in a bathtub. Your surgeon will let you know what your restrictions are and for how long. When you can return to work depends on the operation you had and also the type of work you do.

After most operations, you can have sexual activity when you feel you are able, usually after your stitches or staples are removed.

Normally, you can take a shower after the second postoperative day. Do not soak in the bathtub until your stitches, staples, or Steri-Strips® are removed.

After small-incision procedures, your surgeon may not put a limit on any activities. Resume your activities gradually as pain allows.

If you have a drain in one of your incisions, your surgeon will remove it once the drainage stops.

Even after minor procedures with anesthesia, you should not drive until the anesthetic is out of your system. This process can take 24 hours.

It is easy to overdo after a surgical procedure. Slowly increase your physical activity. Try to do a little more every day. And get plenty of rest.

WHEN SHOULD YOU SEE YOUR SURGEON?

Your surgeon will let you know when she or he expects to see you back

INSIDER'S TIP ▶

Be prepared for the postoperative blues. Feeling down or sad after an operation is common. There is often a letdown after all the energy devoted to coping with the stress of a surgical procedure. Plus, you may hurt and not be able to sleep well. You may feel vulnerable. Or you may have a sense of loss about your health or your appearance (because of a scar, for example). Worry about finances can be an added cause of anxiety at this time.

Talk to friends and family about your fears and feelings during this difficult time. It also helps to have realistic expectations before you have the operation.

Most people cope well with the emotions arising from having an operation. Sometimes, however, patients become depressed. Postoperative depression occurs more often after the patient is home or back at work, rather than right after an operation.

Depression needs to be treated. If you feel sad or depressed for longer than two weeks or you are having thoughts of hurting yourself, tell your doctor. You may need an antidepressant or psychotherapy (talk therapy).

in the office. Typically the first postoperative visit is seven to 10 days after the operation.

This visit is a good time to ask your surgeon about any questions or concerns you may have. But you don't have to wait until then to seek advice. Call your surgeon or a member of the surgeon's staff if you need a question answered between visits.

Less often, the surgeon may not need to see the patient again after the operation. This may be the case if the procedure was minor and there is no need to remove sutures. Or if you live far away from your surgeon, arrangements may be made for you to get postoperative care from a local doctor. You may be asked to keep in touch with the surgeon by phone. Find out if the surgeon's practice uses e-mail.

WHEN WILL YOUR STITCHES COME OUT?

The surgeon usually removes sutures (stitches) during the first or second postoperative visit. The time when sutures come out depends on where on the body the incision is and how quickly the wound heals. It can range from a few days to a few weeks.

Some patients will not need to have their stitches removed, because their surgeon used sutures that dissolve. A surgeon may use dissolvable (absorbable) sutures deep in the wound and then close the skin edges using strips of sterile adhesive tape called Steri-Strips®. These small bandages should be left on until they fall off by themselves. Sometimes Steri-Strips® are used alone without sutures if a wound is not deep.

Surgical staples are another common type of skin closure. Your surgeon will remove them at a postoperative visit or in the hospital days after the operation.

Usually suture or staple removal causes only discomfort or mild pain. But if you are sensitive to pain, you may want to take pain medicine shortly before your surgeon removes the staples or stitches.

Protect the newly healed skin on your surgical site from the sun. New skin burns easily.

WILL YOU NEED OTHER TREATMENTS?

Sometimes other treatment is necessary after a surgical procedure. Cancer patients, for instance, may need chemotherapy or radiation treatment. To give the patient a chance to heal, chemotherapy and radiation therapy generally are not started until three or four weeks after the operation to remove the cancer.

Rehabilitation, such as physical or occupational therapy, often is needed after an orthopedic surgical procedure and sometimes after other procedures. Rehab may begin soon after an operation. Some patients may need to stay at a rehab facility, but often rehab can be done on an outpatient basis.

Sometimes, especially in diabetic patients, a surgical wound does not heal. In such cases, the patient may need treatment from a wound care specialist. Proper healing of the wound is critical to a good surgical result.

WHAT WILL YOU NEED AT HOME TO HAVE A SMOOTH RECOVERY?

At home, you'll need an environment that contributes to healing, where you can get rest and proper nutrition. Your home also should be safe, and you should eliminate things that might cause you to fall. In addition, you may need special equipment or home health care.

A PATIENT'S PERSPECTIVE

Linda Copeland, 59-year-old who had a lumpectomy for treatment of breast cancer 19 years ago, followed by radiation treatment and chemotherapy

"When I found out I had cancer, I thought I was going to die. I chose my surgeon based on his willingness to do a lumpectomy. I was glad I could keep my breast. But sometimes accompanying treatments are more devastating than the operation. One of the most devastating things for me was when the oncologist told me I was going into menopause at age 40 because of chemo. I didn't meet with a medical oncologist before the operation, and no one had mentioned that possibility to me before. Losing my hair after chemo also was [distressing].

"I relied on my faith in God. A positive attitude and a support team are key to a successful recovery, no matter what kind of surgery you have. I also take good care of my health, and I get my annual checkup and screenings. Nineteen years after my operation, I've had no recurrence of cancer."

Special Equipment or Help

Ask your surgeon before you get home if you will need anything special. For example, older patients or those who have had major operations may need a portable bedside toilet, a raised toilet seat, or a bed with a head that can be raised.

In some cases, you may need an assistant or home health care aide for help with certain tasks, such as bathing. You may need a home health (visiting) nurse. You usually will know ahead of time if you will need home health care.

Prevent Falls

Make sure that your home is safe and that you have gotten rid of anything that might cause you to fall. Taking precautions is especially important if you are elderly, taking medicine that makes you groggy or dizzy, or using a walker or crutches. Here are some ways to prevent falls:

- Remove throw rugs or fasten them down with adhesive tape.

- Keep walkways and stairs free of clutter and electrical cords.

- Put a grab bar near the bathtub or shower, or ask for help from a family member while getting in and out of the bath. Also use a nonskid bath mat in the shower or tub.

- When you walk, wear shoes or slippers with soles that are not slippery.

- Keep things you use often near you, so you don't have to keep getting up.

- Improve lighting in dimly lit areas.

- At night, turn on a nightlight in your bathroom.

WILL THERE BE ANY LONG-TERM EFFECTS?

Ask your surgeon if the operation will involve any permanent or long-term changes or side effects. Some operations may mean you will have a permanent change in your activities or function. For instance, doctors may recommend that people not run or perform other high-impact sports after having a knee or hip replaced. Other procedures (for example, organ transplants or thyroid removal) may require lifelong drug treatment. Still other operations, such as removal of part of the intestine, may change bowel function.

HOW BIG WILL YOUR SCAR BE?

Nearly all surgical wounds will leave a scar. A scar is a natural part of healing. With time, your scar will fade somewhat.

The size of the incision, and thus the scar, will depend on whether the operation is performed through a scope using tiny incisions, or a traditional open operation. The incision size also depends on the kind of operation and what area of the body is operated on.

Scar Revision

You may be concerned if your scar is in an obvious area, such as on your face, or in a spot that may restrict movement, such as on a joint. In some people, the scar becomes abnormally raised or sunken. If you are unhappy with the appearance of your scar after it has completely healed, talk to your surgeon. There are medical and surgical ways to flatten a scar or otherwise make it less noticeable. This process is called scar revision. There is no way, however, to completely remove a scar.

Vitamin E Myth

Some people claim that rubbing vitamin E cream on scars helps heal them or improves their cosmetic appearance. However, a study published in 1999 in the journal *Dermatologic Surgery* showed that in most people vitamin E cream did not help improve scars or made them worse. In addition, vitamin E cream caused a rash in one-third of the patients studied. An earlier study also found no benefit to topical vitamin E in reducing scar formation after reconstructive operations.

At this time, there is no scientific evidence to recommend vitamin E use on scars.

WHEN CAN YOU EXPECT TO BE FULLY RECOVERED?

As you probably now understand, having a surgical procedure and recovering from it is not a quick fix to your problem. It will take a while before you feel well again and are back to your normal routine. Full recovery from a major operation could take months to a year. For minor procedures or minimally invasive operations, recovery may take just weeks.

Ask your surgeon what length of recovery to expect. Remember that this time frame is an estimate. Everyone is different. If it takes longer than expected, be patient.

Congratulations!

When your healing is done, congratulate yourself! As an informed patient and an active participant in your surgical process, you have played an important part in your recovery.

As we come to the end of this book, my wish for you is a superb result of your operation and an excellent, trusting relationship with your surgeon and the health care team.

Because this book has been all about you—the patient—I want to close with the words of a patient. Dave Davis shares the wisdom he gained from having a surgical procedure: "Before my operation, I took my health for granted. My operation gave me an awareness of how to take care of myself. Since then, I have made my health more of a priority."

It is clear that making healthy and informed decisions can have a huge impact on any patient's life. If you take care of your health, you may be able to avoid developing certain health problems in the future that could require you to have an operation.

I hope that what you have learned in this book will help you take charge of your health, not just for your upcoming operation, but through-out your lifetime. We are all in this effort together!

What to Ask the Surgeon

☐ What about pain relief?

☐ What should I do about bleeding or other problems?

☐ When can I resume normal activities?

☐ When should I next see my surgeon?

☐ When will my stitches come out?

☐ Will I need other treatments?

☐ What will I need at home to have a smooth recovery?

☐ Will there be any long-term effects?

☐ How big will my scar be?

☐ When can I expect to be fully recovered?

Glossary

abdomen: What you usually call your stomach. To your doctor, it refers to the digestive, urinary, and reproductive organs in the cavity from the diaphragm to the pelvis.

ABMS: American Board of Medical Specialties. The not-for-profit organization that oversees certification of physicians in their specialties.

absorbable suture: Suture that dissolves.

accreditation: Credential showing that a health care facility has met high standards for performance and safety.

acute: Severe and short-term, not chronic (as in an illness).

adhesion: Fibrous band of scar tissue that can form anytime after an abdominal operation. It can bind organs or other internal body structures.

admitting privileges: Physician's right to admit patients to a hospital.

adrenal gland: Pair of glands on the kidneys that produce hormones that control important functions, such as blood pressure, heart rate, and the body's response to stress.

advance directive: Legal document to be used for health care decisions when someone cannot speak for himself or herself. See living will and power of attorney for health care.

adverse: Unfavorable, unwanted, as in effects of a drug or complications of a procedure.

altruism: Unselfishness; dedication to others' well-being.

ambulatory: Outpatient, as in ambulatory surgical facility.

analgesia: Pain relief.

analgesic: Medicine that relieves pain.

anemic: Having an abnormally low number of red blood cells. Sometimes called iron-poor blood.

anesthesia: Use of a substance (gas, injection, paste, or liquid) to remove sensitivity to pain. The substance is called an anesthetic. A physician who performs anesthesia is called an anesthesiologist. A nurse who is certified to perform anesthesia is a nurse anesthetist.

anesthesiologist: Physician who performs anesthesia.

anesthetist: See nurse anesthetist.

angioplasty: Minimally invasive procedure using a balloon to open a blocked or narrowed artery, a blood vessel of the heart. Also called balloon angioplasty.

appendicitis: Infection of the appendix.

appendix: Small, narrow, hollow organ that is part of the large intestine. It has no useful function in humans and occasionally gets infected (appendicitis).

arterial line: Thin catheter inserted into an artery in the wrist or groin to constantly monitor blood pressure or to obtain blood samples for monitoring blood oxygen levels.

artery: Blood vessel that carries blood from the heart to the body.

autologous: Refers to self, as in an autologous blood donation.

bariatric surgical procedure: Weight-loss operation performed in selected patients who are morbidly (very) obese. Types of bariatric procedures include gastric bypass, gastric banding, or "stomach stapling."

benign: Noncancerous.

bilateral: Two-sided. Normally refers to right side and left side.

biopsy: Sampling of tissue from an abnormal area, such as a lump or tumor.

blood transfusion: Replacement of blood lost during an operation or injury.

board-certified: Credential showing that a physician has passed examinations that test knowledge in a specialty of medicine.

bowel obstruction: See intestinal obstruction.

candidate: Patient who is eligible to have a specific treatment or surgical procedure.

cardiopulmonary resuscitation: See CPR.

cardiovascular: Refers to the heart and blood vessels.

cataract: Clouding of the normally clear lens of the eye. The lens helps the eye to focus.

CT scan: Computed tomography. A huge machine that takes multiple X-rays of the body at short intervals. A computer then integrates these X-rays to give precise images of the body, bones, internal organs, or brain. A special computer program can make the images three-dimensional. Used widely for diagnosis and to observe disease, such as cancerous tumors, during treatment. Sometimes called CAT scan (computed axial tomography).

catheter: Tube that comes in various sizes and is used to inject fluids or medicines, and to remove blood and other body fluids.

chaplain: A clergy member or other faith leader who meets the religious and spiritual needs of patients in a hospital.

charge nurse: The nurse leader on the inpatient floor who is responsible for overall care, planning, staffing, and operations. Usually this nurse is very experienced and has no direct patient care assignment.

chemotherapy: Multiple medicines used singly or in combination to treat cancer and sometimes other diseases. May be called "chemo."

chronic: Ongoing, long-term medical condition.

clinical nurse specialist: Registered nurse with advanced education and training in one area of nursing.

clinical trial: Research study that tests a new treatment in people or compares two or more existing treatments.

complication: An unexpected and unwanted result of a medical treatment or surgical procedure. Differs from a side effect, which is an unwanted effect expected to happen sometimes. A side effect can lead to a complication.

compression stockings: Long tight socks worn to put pressure on the leg muscles, to avoid a blood clot forming after an operation.

conscious sedation: Use of sedatives and pain medicine in which the patient stays awake but probably will not remember the procedure.

constipation: Difficulty in passing stool, or hard or infrequent stools.

CPR: Cardiopulmonary resuscitation. A lifesaving procedure of rescue breaths and chest compressions to restore someone's breathing after the heart stops.

critical care unit: See intensive care unit.

dietitian: Person trained in nutrition.

differential diagnosis: List of possible diagnoses to explain symptoms.

discharge: Doctor's order that a patient is ready to go home from a hospital or surgical facility.

durable power of attorney for health care: See power of attorney for health care.

Echocardiogram (ECG or EKG): An ultrasonogram (ultrasound image) of the heart. Shows shadows of the heart chambers, valves, and major blood vessels. With the addition of color, it shows the direction of blood flow in all parts of the heart.

elective operation: Planned operation, which is not needed right away but scheduled at a convenient time for the surgeon and the patient.

electrocardiogram: A test that records the electrical activity of the heart. Measures the rate and regularity of heart beats, the size and position of the chambers, presence of damage to the heart, and the effects of drugs or devices (like a pacemaker) to regulate the heart.

emergency surgical procedure: Operation that must be done soon after symptoms of an acute condition begin. Usually it is within hours of a diagnosis.

endoscope: Small lighted viewing tube similar to a telescope, used to see inside the body during a minimally invasive procedure.

ER: Emergency room. Area in the hospital where emergency conditions are first treated. Also called emergency department (ED).

esophagus: Part of the digestive canal between the throat and stomach, through which food passes.

FACS: Fellow of the American College of Surgeons. Designation for members of the College.

fast-track surgery: Although this term or concept isn't used everywhere, it means a surgical approach that uses a combination of techniques to reduce the body's stress response and to shorten recovery time. Also called rapid recovery.

fellowship: Training program after residency to gain experience in a medical or surgical specialty or subspecialty.

fibroid: Benign tumor, sometimes found in the uterus (womb).

gallbladder: Organ beneath the liver that stores bile, a substance that helps in the digestion of fats.

gastrointestinal: Refers to the stomach and intestine.

general anesthesia: Patient is asleep. Major operations usually are performed this way. It often is started with an intravenous (IV) drug and then maintained with a gas, requiring the patient to breathe through a mask or tube.

general surgeon: Surgeon who is trained in the diagnosis and management of a broad range of surgical conditions.

hernia: Protrusion of tissue in the abdominal wall. See inguinal hernia.

HIPAA: Health Insurance Portability and Accountability Act. This 1996 federal law requires most health care organizations to supply you with a privacy notice, which explains the organization's practices of how it uses your health information and how it keeps identifying information confidential.

hospitalist: Hospital-based doctor specially trained to take care of patients in the hospital.

hysterectomy: Removal of the uterus (womb).

ICU: See intensive care unit.

ileus: See paralytic ileus.

incentive spirometer: A device used by the patient after an operation for breathing exercises that help expand the lungs and prevent lung complications.

incision: Cut made in the skin and tissues to perform a surgical procedure.

incontinence: Inability to control one's bladder (urinary incontinence) or bowel (fecal incontinence).

induction: Usually refers to the initial process of anesthesia. May also be used for the first treatment with cancer medicines, as in chemotherapy induction.

informed consent: Process of giving written permission to have a procedure and indicating that one understands why the procedure is needed, its intended result, and its risks and benefits.

infusion pump: Intravenous pump used to give IV fluids and drugs.

inguinal hernia: Hernia (protrusion of tissue) occurring in the groin (inguinal region), the area between the top of the thigh and the lowest part of the belly.

injection: Shot of medicine or fluids into the body by a needle or needle system. See entries for intravenous (IV) and intramuscular.

intensive care unit: Special unit of the hospital where patients receive close monitoring and extra care. Also called ICU or critical care unit.

intensivist: Doctor specially trained to take care of critically ill patients in the hospital and who coordinates care with the patient's surgeon and primary care doctor.

intern: Physician in the first postgraduate year of training after graduating from medical school. Also known as PGY-1, postgraduate year one.

intestine: Tube-like structure in the body that aids in digestion, provides the body with water and nutrients, and moves stool. Also called bowel and gut.

intestinal obstruction: Blockage of the intestine. Symptoms include stomach pain, bloating, and vomiting. Also called bowel obstruction.

intraocular lens: Artificial lens implanted in the eye to substitute for the natural lens, which is partly or totally removed during a cataract operation.

intraoperative awareness: See surgical awareness.

intramuscular: Means "inside a muscle." May refer to an injection into a muscle or to describe the location of something abnormal. Example: an intramuscular mass.

intravenous (IV): Way of putting fluids or medications into a vein, usually with a small plastic tube or catheter.

intubation: Insertion of a tube, such as a catheter, into the body.

invasive surgical procedure: Surgical procedure that involves cutting or puncturing the skin or insertion of surgical instruments into the body.

Joint Commission: The national organization that oversees accreditation of many health care facilities.

kidney: One of two organs that are part of the urinary system.

laparoscopy: See minimally invasive surgery.

licensed practical nurse (LPN), licensed vocational nurse (LVN): A person licensed by the state to do certain basic levels of patient care at the bedside. Reports to a registered nurse.

liver: Organ that helps in digestion and cleanses the blood.

living will: Written record of the health care an individual requests if that person is unable to make his or her own medical decisions.

local anesthesia: Numbing of a small area of skin and tissue under the skin so that a painless cut can be made. Can be applied to the skin as a paste or shot. The injection hurts a little as the needle goes in, then numbs the area of injection. Pain loss lasts from 30 minutes to two hours depending on the numbing medicine used. Often used for minor outpatient procedures.

lumpectomy: Removal of a cancerous breast tumor and a small area of tissue around it.

lymph gland: Swelling of tissue in the lymphatic system, a lymph gland traps tumors and infections. Often enlarges with infection—for example, in the throat, ear, or eye, or in cases where the cancer spreads to it. The lymphatic system, also called lymphatics, is a system of colorless vessels running throughout the body. The lymphatics gather up tissue fluids and return them through larger channels to a vein in the neck. Also called lymph node.

lymph node: See lymph gland.

magnetic resonance imaging: See MRI.

major surgical procedure: Operation that requires anesthesia or respiratory assistance.

malignant: Cancerous, as when cells have the capacity to grow outside of the place they began and spread to other parts of the body by direct growth, bloodstream, or the lymphatic system. May require an operation, chemotherapy, radiation treatment, or a combination of these therapies to control or halt the cancer. There are many types of malignant tumors.

mastectomy: Removal of an entire breast, usually because of breast cancer.

medical durable power of attorney: See power of attorney for health care.

medical student: Person who after college attends medical school. Spends the first two years of medical school in classes and laboratories and the last two years on clinical rotations in hospitals. The medical degree (MD) is awarded on graduation. Graduates of an osteopathic medical school earn a DO (doctor of osteopathy).

minimally invasive surgery: Technique in which a surgeon does a deep surgical procedure by passing long-handled instruments through several tiny incisions. A video image of the inside of the body, taken by a small camera inserted into the body, enlarges the surgical area and allows the surgeon to see what she is doing. Laparoscopy is an operation in the abdomen; thoracoscopy, a surgical procedure in the chest.

minor surgical procedure: An operation that is less invasive, of short duration (usually less than an hour), and has a shorter period of recovery. A minor procedure does not require general anesthesia or respiratory assistance.

MRI: Magnetic resonance imaging. Technique that shows images of the internal parts of the body but does not use X-rays. The machine is a large magnet that acts on the millions of magnets in the human body, lining them up. A computer interprets these images and presents them as an internal image of the body. Often used for imaging bones, tumors, and the brain and spinal cord.

narcotic: Prescription painkiller, such as morphine, codeine, or oxycodone.

negative: Normal, as in the result of a lab test or biopsy.

NSAID: Nonsteroidal anti-inflammatory drug, such as ibuprofen or naproxen. Relieves pain and inflammation.

nurse anesthetist: Registered nurse who is certified to perform anesthesia.

nurse practitioner: Advanced practice nurse with a master's degree and special training. Can practice in an inpatient setting, outpatient setting, or both. Often functions as a physician extender. This varies from state to state, from full independence to practicing with a physician.

nurse's aide: A patient care assistant in the hospital who is not a registered nurse. Also called nurse assistant.

occupational therapist: Person trained to help patients acquire or reacquire life skills, such as feeding, dressing, and bathing.

oncologist: Doctor who specializes in the treatment of cancer.

oncology: The study of cancer.

open surgical technique: Manner of performing an operation in which the surgeon makes a cut in the body. (Differs from a minimally invasive surgical procedure.)

operating room (OR): Room in which an operation is performed.

opioid: Morphine-like narcotic medication used to reduce pain.

orthopedic surgeon: Physician with extensive training in the diagnosis and treatment, both nonsurgical and surgical, of the musculoskeletal system, including muscles, bones, joints, ligaments (tissues connecting bones), tendons (tissues connecting muscles to bones), and nerves.

outcome: Result, such as of an operation.

over-the-counter: Available without a doctor's prescription, as in medication.

oxygen saturation: Percentage that shows how well the lungs provide oxygen to the blood. It is the percentage of hemoglobin (the oxygen-transporting protein in red blood cells) in the blood.

PACU: Postanesthesia care unit. See recovery room.

pancreas: Solid organ in the mid-upper abdomen. It makes enzymes to digest food, which empty through a duct, a hollow tube, into the duodenum (see intestine). It also makes insulin, which controls blood sugar.

paralytic ileus: Temporary intestinal paralysis (inability to move the bowels) that can occur after an abdominal operation.

patient-controlled analgesia: See PCA.

patient liaison: In a hospital, the person who helps patients and their families resolve nonmedical problems, such as complaints about the facility, quality of care, or access to care. May be called patient representative.

patient-to-nurse ratio: Number of patients that each hospital floor nurse cares for.

PCA: Patient-controlled analgesia. An intravenous device that allows the patient to push a button and release pain medications into the bloodstream. The dose is carefully calculated, and there is a "lockout" mechanism on the machine so the patient cannot overdose.

phlebotomist: Health professional trained to draw blood for testing.

physical therapist: Rehabilitation professional who evaluates and treats movement dysfunction; for example, teaches walking with crutches and retrains muscles that have lost function from an operation or injury.

physical therapy: Rehabilitation to restore function and independence.

physician's assistant: Person licensed by the state to perform the functions of a physician extender. This person is usually not a nurse so does not have a nurse's breadth of medical knowledge. Practices under the supervision of a physician.

plastic surgeon: Physician with special training in performing cosmetic and reconstructive surgery.

pneumonia: Lung infection.

postanesthesia care unit: See recovery room.

postoperative: After an operation.

power of attorney for health care: Legal document stating who will make decisions about a person's medical care if that person becomes incapacitated. Also called medical durable power of attorney.

preauthorization: Required advance notice to an insurer that a member of the insurance plan is having major treatment such as a hospital admission. Also called precertification.

preemptive pain control: Medical pain relief given before an operation, to try to preempt, or forestall, pain after the procedure. Not used very frequently.

preoperative: Before an operation.

preregistration: Process of giving a surgical facility insurance and medical information before the day of an operation. Also called preadmission.

prophylaxis: Preventive treatment, as in antibiotic prophylaxis.

prostate: Male gland that works with the bladder muscles to control urine flow. It also contributes to the fluid in semen.

prostatectomy: Removal of the prostate.

pulse oximeter: A device, typically put on a fingertip, that measures oxygen saturation.

radiation therapy: Strong X-ray beams are directed at the area to be treated, such as a cancerous tumor. This technique involves sophisticated methods of outlining the tumor, gauging its size, and determining how much radiation is needed to shrink the tumor. May be used in combination with chemotherapy and an operation.

radiologist: Doctor who is in charge of the equipment used for imaging diagnostic tests, including ultrasound, X-ray, CT, MRI, and PET. Also reads the images produced. Radiology is a medical specialty and requires years of study after medical school.

recovery room: Place where the patient spends time to awaken from anesthesia. Also called postanesthesia care unit (PACU). How long you spend there depends on, among other things, the length of your operation and the anesthesia you received.

regional anesthesia: Injection of a local anesthetic into the nerves supplying the area to be numbed. It takes longer to act than a local anesthetic but lasts longer. Used when a larger area needs numbing.

registered nurse: Person who is trained to plan and give patient care. May be trained in a two-year school and hold a diploma or may have a bachelor's or master's degree in nursing. Is licensed by the state, which develops and monitors standards. See also nurse practitioner.

resection: Removal of all or part of an organ or other structure.

residency: Postmedical school training program in a medical or surgical specialty, such as general surgery. Length of the training program varies by specialty.

resident: Graduate of a medical school who is training in a medical or surgical specialty. Also called house staff.

respirator: A machine that takes over breathing when a patient cannot breathe on his own or struggles to breathe. The machine pumps oxygen into the lungs through a tube in the windpipe. Also called ventilator.

respiratory therapist: Person who is licensed to deal with patients' airways and breathing machines. Works with the nurses and physicians but cannot practice alone and cannot give intravenous medications. Can give inhalant medications with a physician order. Seen in an intensive care unit where patients are on breathing machines.

rule out: Exclusion of a diagnosis. For example, "rule out appendicitis" means it is not clear if the patient has appendicitis. The rule out label disappears once the doctor makes the diagnosis.

second opinion: Opinion from a second physician about the patient's diagnosis and recommended medical treatment.

sedative: Medication that makes a patient calm, often sleepy. Procedures can be performed under sedation without agitating or hurting the patient, who will not remember having anything done.

sinus: Space next to the nasal passage, which can become infected (sinusitis).

social worker: Professional who works to enhance the social functioning of the patient and the patient's family. The hospital's clinical social worker may help with preadmission and discharge planning, give psychosocial or financial counseling, lead support groups, follow up with a patient after discharge, or connect the patient with community resources.

speech therapist: Rehab professional who evaluates and treats patients who have problems swallowing, talking, or thinking.

Spinal anesthesia (epidural): Injection of local anesthesia (or morphine for pain control) into the back between the bones of the spine. May be used alone with the patient awake or sedated, or to supplement general anesthesia. Spinal anesthesia works well for pain control after an operation; in this case, the tube used to administer the anesthetic may be left in for a few days.

spinal fusion: Joining together the vertebrae (the bony segments of the spine) above and below where a damaged disc (a "shock absorber" that cushions the vertebrae) was removed.

Steri-Strip: Brand name for a type of adhesive skin closure strip.

steroid: Type of drug that reduces inflammation and swelling or increases low amounts of the male hormone testosterone. Anabolic (type of steroid) refers to muscle building.

subspecialty: Specialized area within a medical or surgical specialty. Spine surgery, for example, is a subspecialty under orthopedic surgery.

surgical awareness: Unexpected awakening during a surgical procedure using general anesthesia (a rare occurrence).

surgical intervention: Surgical treatment; surgical procedure.

surgical site: Area of the body that is or was operated on.

surgical-site infection: An infection of the surgical wound or any organ or body space entered during the operation.

suture: Surgical stitch used to close an incision.

teaching hospital: Hospital where, under the supervision of trained physicians, medical students learn to become physicians and where physicians train in their chosen specialty as surgical residents.

thoracoscopy: See minimally invasive surgery.

time-out: Surgical time-out refers to the final safety check in the operating room before the operation begins. Its purpose is to ensure the correct operation in the correct patient.

tonsillectomy: Operation to remove the tonsils.

topical anesthetic: Local anesthetic (numbing medicine) applied to the skin as an ointment or spray.

triage: Process of deciding how urgent a condition is and how immediate treatment needs to be. Used in an emergency room.

tumor: Lump or abnormal growth, which may be benign or malignant.

ultrasound: Machine that generates sound waves which are bounced off internal organs and projected onto a screen as shadows. These can be used to check normal and diseased organs.

urinary catheter: Tube inserted through a female patient's urinary tract into the bladder or attached to a male's penis. Used to collect urine into a bag.

uterine: Refers to the uterus, or womb.

vascular: Refers to blood vessels.

veins: Blood vessels that carry the blood back to the heart. They contain blood without much oxygen and therefore look blue.

ventilator: See respirator.

vital organ: Organ in the body that is essential for life, such as the heart.

vital signs: Physical signs that someone is alive, such as blood pressure, temperature, pulse, heartbeat, and breathing rate.

wrong-site surgical procedure: An operation that is performed on the wrong side or area of a patient's body (a rare occurrence).

X ray: An invisible beam of energy that goes through flesh and produces images on a special screen.

APPENDIX A

About the American College of Surgeons

The American College of Surgeons is the largest organization of surgeons in the world. It is a scientific and educational association that was founded in 1913 to improve the quality of care for the surgical patient by setting high standards for surgical education and practice.

Patient education is an important service provided by the College. Through its patient education Web site, "Patients as Partners in Surgical Care" (www.facs.org/patienteducation/index.html), and its brochure series on frequently performed surgical procedures, the College provides the public with information to help them make informed decisions about surgical care.

MEMBERSHIP

Surgeons who are members of the American College of Surgeons are known as Fellows. The letters "FACS" after a surgeon's name mean Fellow, American College of Surgeons. These letters indicate that the surgeon's education and training, professional qualifications, surgical competence, and ethical conduct passed a rigorous evaluation and met the high standards of the College.

The College has more than 72,000 Fellows, including more than 6,000 Fellows in other countries.

The American College of Surgeons seal was designed in 1915 and has been in use ever since. It shows Aesculapius, the Greek symbol of medicine and healing, and an American Indian medicine man. Both sit beneath a tree of knowledge, offering their symbols of healing in common service to mankind. The Latin words at the bottom of the seal, *Omnibus per artem fidemque prodesse,* mean "To serve all with skill and fidelity."

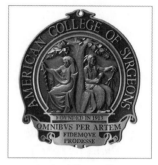

Seal of the College

OTHER PUBLICATIONS FROM THE ACS

Public Information Brochures on Frequently Performed Operations

About Appendectomy (Surgical removal of the appendix)

About Low Back Pain (Surgical intervention to treat a variety of common conditions that cause low back pain)

About Carotid Endarterectomy (Surgical removal of blockages from blood vessels in the neck)

About Cataract Surgery in Adults (Surgical removal of cataracts to improve vision)

About Cesarean Section (Delivery of a baby through a surgical incision in the mother's lower abdominal wall and uterus)

About Cholecystectomy (Surgical removal of the gallbladder)

About D&C for Miscarriage (A surgical procedure performed to scrape the internal lining of the uterus following miscarriage)

About D&C for Uterine Bleeding Problems (A surgical procedure performed to scrape the internal lining of the uterus to diagnose and treat abnormal uterine bleeding)

About Hernia Repair (Surgical repair of hernias)

About Hysteroscopy (Examination of the interior uterus to diagnose or treat uterine problems)

About Hysterectomy (Surgical removal of organs in the female reproductive system)

About Prostatectomy (for BPH) (Surgical removal of all, or parts of, the prostate)

About Tonsillectomy and Adenoidectomy (Surgical removal of the tonsils and adenoids)

These brochures are available for free downloading at www.facs.org/public_ info/operation/aboutbroch.html. Or you can order a single copy at no charge by calling the American College of Surgeons at 312-202-5391.

APPENDIX B

Surgical Specialties

CARDIOTHORACIC SURGERY: Surgery of the chest and heart

Certifying Board*: American Board of Thoracic Surgery

Subspecialties†: Certificate: Congenital heart surgery (available in 2007 or 2008)

COLON AND RECTAL SURGERY: Surgery of the intestinal tract, colon, rectum, anus

Certifying Board*: American Board of Colon and Rectal Surgery

GENERAL SURGERY: Treatment of a broad range of surgical conditions affecting many areas of the body

Certifying Board*: American Board of Surgery

Subspecialties†: Certificates: Hand surgery; pediatric surgery; surgical critical care; vascular surgery

NEUROLOGICAL SURGERY: Treatment of disorders of the nervous system, which includes the spinal column, spinal cord, brain, and peripheral nerves (nerves outside the brain and spinal cord)

Certifying Board*: American Board of Neurological Surgery

OBSTETRICS AND GYNECOLOGY: Treatment of conditions that affect the female reproductive system; medical and surgical care for pregnant women; and delivery of babies

Certifying Board*: American Board of Obstetrics and Gynecology

Subspecialties†: Certificates: Gynecologic oncology; maternal and fetal medicine; reproductive endocrinology/infertility. Other subspecialty: Female pelvic medicine and reconstruction

111

OPHTHALMIC SURGERY: Surgery to treat diseases and injuries of the eyes and to correct or restore vision

CERTIFYING BOARD*: AMERICAN BOARD OF OPHTHALMOLOGY

Subspecialties†: Cataract/anterior segment surgery; cornea/external (eye) disease surgery; glaucoma; neuro-ophthalmology; oculoplastics; pediatric ophthalmology/ strabismus surgery; refractive management; retina/vitreous surgery; uveitis

ORTHOPEDIC SURGERY: Surgery of the musculoskeletal system: bones, joints, muscles, associated nerves, arteries, and overlying skin

Certifying Board*: American Board of Orthopaedic Surgery

Subspecialties†: Certificates: Hand surgery; orthopedic sports medicine. Other subspecialties: Foot and ankle orthopedics; joint replacement; pediatric orthopedics; orthopedic oncology; orthopedic trauma surgery; spine surgery

OTOLARYNGOLOGY-HEAD AND NECK SURGERY: Surgery of the ear, nose, and throat (ENT), including the respiratory system and the mouth, esophagus, and stomach

Certifying Board*: American Board of Otolaryngology

Subspecialties†: Certificates: Head and neck plastic surgery; neurotology (ear surgery); pediatric otolaryngology; sleep medicine

PEDIATRIC SURGERY: Surgery in children and teenagers

Certifying Board*: American Board of Surgery

PLASTIC SURGERY: Reconstruction of facial and body defects; cosmetic enhancement of appearance

Certifying Board*: American Board of Plastic Surgery

Subspecialties†: Certificate: Hand surgery. Other subspecialty: Head and neck plastic surgery

UROLOGICAL SURGERY: Treatment of medical and surgical disorders of the adrenal gland and genital-urinary systems

Certifying Board*: American Board of Urology

Subspecialties†: Pediatric urology

VASCULAR SURGERY: Treatment of diseases that affect the arteries and veins throughout the body

Certifying Board*: American Board of Surgery

* Member boards of the American Board of Medical Specialties.

† Some boards have subspecialty certificates that members of the specialty may earn. Other boards offer no subspecialty certificates, but the specialty has recognized subspecialty areas in which members may receive additional training, such as a fellowship, or limit their scope of practice.

APPENDIX C

Surgical Specialty Organizations

Organization*	Website	Address/Phone
American College of Surgeons	www.facs.org	633 N. Saint Clair St. Chicago, IL 60611-3211 Phone: 312-202-5000
American Academy of Ophthalmology	www.aao.org	PO Box 7424 San Francisco, CA 94120 Phone: 415-561-8500
American Academy of Orthopaedic Surgeons	www.aaos.org	6300 N. River Rd. Rosemont, IL 60018 Phone: 847-823-7186
American Academy of Otolaryngology—Head and Neck Surgery	www.aaohns.org	1 Prince St. Alexandria, VA 22314 Phone: 703-836-4444
American Association of Neurological Surgeons	www.neurosurgery today.org	5550 Meadowbrook Dr. Rolling Meadows, IL 60008 Phone: 888-566-AANS (2267)
American College of Obstetricians and Gynecologists	www.acog.org	409 12th St., SW P.O. Box 96920 Washington, DC 20090 Phone: 202-638-5577

ORGANIZATION*	WEBSITE	ADDRESS/PHONE
American Pediatric Surgical Association	www.eapsa.org	60 Revere Dr., Suite 500 Northbrook, IL 60062 Phone: 847-480-9576
American Society of Colon and Rectal Surgeons	www.fascrs.org	85 W. Algonquin Rd., Suite 550 Arlington Heights, IL 60005 Phone: 847-290-9184
American Society of Plastic Surgeons	www.plasticsurgery.org	444 E. Algonquin Rd. Arlington Heights, IL 60005 Phone: 888-4PLASTIC (475-2784)
American Urological Association	www.urologyhealth.org	1000 Corporate Boulevard Linthicum, MD 21090 Phone: 866-RING AUA (746-4282)
Society of Thoracic Surgeons	www.sts.org	633 N. Saint Clair St., Suite 2320 Chicago, IL 60611 Phone: 312-202-5800
Society for Vascular Surgery	www.vascularweb.org	633 N. Saint Clair St., 24th Floor Chicago, IL 60611 Phone: 800-258-7188

U.S. surgical specialty organizations recognized by the American College of Surgeons.

OTHER SURGICAL AND RELATED ORGANIZATIONS

American Board of Medical Specialties • www.abms.org

American Association of Nurse Anesthetists • www.anesthesiapatientsafety.com

American Society of Anesthesiologists • www.asahq.org

American Society of Transplant Surgeons • www.asts.org

Society of Critical Care Medicine • www.sccm.org

Index

A

accreditation, of surgical facilities,
 13–14, 30–31, 93
Accreditation Association for
 Ambulatory Health Care, 13
ACS. *See* American College of
 Surgeons (ACS)
activities, return to normal, 85
admitting process, 49–52
advance directives, 44–45, 93
alcohol, avoiding after operation, 82
American Association for
 Accreditation of Ambulatory
 Surgical Facilities, 13
American Board of Medical
 Specialties (ABMS), and
 certification, 12–13, 15, 93
American Cancer Society, treatment
 options, 26
American College of Surgeons (ACS),
 107–109
 Code of Professional Conduct, 14,
 20–22
 Commission on Cancer, 14
 Fellowship in, 14, 15

on informed consent, 32
 locating surgeons, 16
 Oncology Group, 27
 and patient education, 6, 26,
 108–109
 on payment, 47
 on surgical site marking, 53–55
American Osteopathic Association, 13
anesthesia, 37–40, 56, 94
appetite loss, after operation, 83

B

bed rest, 70, 75
benefits of operation, 27
Bill of Rights, for patients, 9–10
billing, for operation, 47–48
bleeding, at home, 83, 84
blood clots, preventing, 57, 70
blood transfusions, 31, 43–44, 95
breathing difficulty, at home, 83

C

cancer care
 choosing facility, 13–14
 clinical trials and, 26, 27, 95

treatments after operation, 87-88
chest pain, at home, 83
children, and operations, 32, 108
clinical trials, discussing with
    surgeon, 26–27
Code of Professional Conduct, for
    ACS Fellows, 14, 20–22
complications
    after operation, 83–84, 95–96
    of operation, 27, 95–96
conscious sedation, 38, 96
consent, informed, 32, 50–51, 98
constipation, after operation, 82–83,
    96
credentials, of surgeons, 12–15

D

dehydration, after operation, 84
depression, after operation, 84, 86
diet, after operation, 76–77, 82–83
discharge from facility, after
    operation, 77–80, 96
doctor-patient relationship, 7–8, 18–22
    See also questions for surgeon.
donating blood, 43–44
drains, removal of, 85
drug use, and surgery risks, 28

E

eating
    after operation, 76–77, 82–83
    before operation, 40, 51
education
    importance for patients, 91
    on medical condition, 6–10
    of surgeons *See* surgeon, choosing
emotional preparation, for operation,
    45–46
equipment, medical, 69–70, 79, 89

F

FACS (Fellow of American College of
    Surgeons), 14, 97
family members, involvement of, 8, 24
fast-track surgery, 60–61, 97
fever, at home, 84
financial concerns, 47–48
fluid retention, after operation, 83

G

general anesthesia, 37–38, 97
glossary, 93–106

H

healing. *See* recovery.
health, improving before surgery,
    28–29
health care providers, 39, 72–73
HIPAA (Health Insurance Portability
    and Accountability Act of 1996),
    51, 97
home health care, 32, 79
hospitals, 13–14, 30–31
    accreditation of, 13–14, 30–31
    billing, 47–48
    health care providers, 72–73
    ICU (intensive care unit), 69–70
    room choice, 65–66
    safety factors, 36–37

I

ICU (intensive care unit), 69–70, 97
infection control, 56–57, 58, 75
infections, 56–58, 75
    signs and symptoms of, 79
informed consent, 32, 50–51, 98
informed patient. *See* education;
    informed consent; questions for
    surgeon.
insurance information, 47–48

J

The Joint Commission
  and accreditation, 13, 99
  and surgical site marking, 54–55

L

length of stay, after operation, 42
living wills, 44–45, 99
local anesthesia, 38, 99

M

managed care, arrangements, 47–48
marking of surgical site, 53–55
medications
  at home, 81–83
  postoperative, 66–69
  preoperative, 38, 41, 52–53
  preventing errors, 73–74

N

narcotics, 67–68, 82–83, 100
normal activities, return to, 85
NSAIDs (non-steroidal anti-
  inflammatory drugs), 67, 82,
  101
nurses, 39, 72, 101, 103

O

The Official ABMS Directory of
  Board Certified Medical
  Specialists, 14
operation
  alternatives to, 8, 25–27
  events during, 56–58
  fast-track surgery, 60–61
  length of, 57–59
  length of stay after, 42
  long-term effects of, 89-90
  necessity of, 24–25
  postoperative events, 32–33,
    58–59
  preoperative events, 31, 50–57
  results and recovery, 27–29
  risks and benefits of, 27
  team members and facility, 30–31
  techniques, 29–30
organizations
  for surgical specialties, 113–114
  See also specific organization.
outcome, improving chances of
  good, 28–29, 46

P

pain, at home, 79, 84
pain relief
  during and after operation, 66–69
  at home, 81–83, 84
Patients' Bill of Rights, 9–10
PCAs (patient-controlled analgesia)
    pumps, 68–69, 102
postoperative events, 32–33, 58–59
  breathing and bowel function,
    70–71
  discharge from facility, 77–80
  early movement, 75
  pain relief, 66–69
  recovery time, 63–65
  resuming diet, 76–77
  visit to surgeon, 86-87
  See also recovery.
power of attorney, 45, 102
preauthorization, for operation, 48,
    102
preoperative events, 28–29, 40–48,
    52–58
  advance directives, 44–45
  emotional preparation, 45–46
  insurance, 47–48
  medications, 52–53
  testing, 31

Q

qualifications, of surgeons, 12–15
questions for surgeon, 6–9
    about results, 22, 27–29
    about surgeon, 22
    after discharge, 92
    basic details about operation, 34
    postoperative concerns, 34,
        58–59, 61, 80
    preoperative concerns, 48, 61

R

recovery, 28, 63–66
    complications after operation,
        83–84, 95–96
    at home, 81–92
    in recovery room, 59, 103
    safe environment for, 88–89
    scars and, 90
    special equipment, 79, 88–89
    See also fast-track surgery; pain
        relief.
referrals
    for community resources, 80
    by physician, 16–17
regional anesthesia, 38, 103
registration and admitting, 49–52
rehabilitation, 78, 87
respirators, after operation, 69, 104
responsibilities, as patient, 6–9
rights, as patient, 6–10
risks of operation, 27

S

safety
    and recovery, 88–89
    of surgical facility, 36–37
scars, 90
second opinion, seeking, 17–18, 104
sexual activities, return to, 85

smoking, 29, 42, 85
special equipment, 79, 88–89
staff, surgical, 30, 36–37
staples, 85, 87
statistics on surgery, 2
Steri-Strips, 85, 87, 105
stitches, 85-87
surgeon, choosing, 11–22
    experience of, 15
    finding qualified, 16–17
    interpersonal skills of, 18–20
    qualifications of, 12–15
    surgical specialties, 111–114
    training of, 11–12
    See also Code of Professional
        Conduct.
surgical facilities, 13–14, 30–31
    safety factors, 36–37
surgical sites, marking of, 53–55
surgical techniques, 29–30
sutures, 85-87, 105

T

time-out, 55, 105
transfusions, 31, 43–44
treatment options, 25–27

U

urinary bladder catheters, 76, 84, 106
US National Institutes of Health,
    clinical trials information, 27

V

ventilators, after operation, 69, 106
Vitamin E, and scars, 90
vomiting, at home, 79

W

work, return to, 85
wound care, 88